CARING WITH VITALITY

Yoga and Wellbeing for Foster Carers, Adopters and Their Families

CARING WITH VITALITY

Yoga and Wellbeing for Foster Carers, Adopters and Their Families

Everyday Ideas to Help You Cope and Thrive!

ANDREA WARMAN AND LIZ LARK

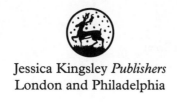

Jessica Kingsley *Publishers*
London and Philadelphia

First published in 2016
by Jessica Kingsley Publishers
73 Collier Street
London N1 9BE, UK
and
400 Market Street, Suite 400
Philadelphia, PA 19106, USA

www.jkp.com

Library of Congress Cataloging in Publication Data
Names: Warman, Andrea, author. | Lark, Liz, author.
Title: Caring with vitality : yoga and wellbeing for foster carers, adopters
    and their families everyday ideas to help you cope and thrive! / Andrea
    Warman and Liz Lark.
Description: Philadelphia : Jessica Kingsley Publishers, 2016. | Includes
    index.
Identifiers: LCCN 2015038792 | ISBN 9781849056649 (alk. paper)
Subjects: LCSH: Caregivers--Psychology. | Yoga--Psychological aspects. |
    Yoga--Social aspects. | Vitality.
Classification: LCC HV41 .W347 2016 | DDC 613.7/046085--dc23 LC record available at
http://lccn.loc.gov/2015038792

British Library Cataloguing in Publication Data
A CIP catalogue record for this book is available from the British Library

ISBN 978 1 84905 664 9
eISBN 978 1 78450 167 9

Printed and bound in Great Britain

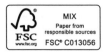

For our mothers, who showed us how to care.

ACKNOWLEDGEMENTS

This book draws on a pilot project, led by authors Andrea and Liz at the ISP Centre in Teynham, Kent, which introduced regular yoga practice and healthy eating to a group of foster carers and evaluated the impact on their health, wellbeing and fostering. The resulting report was published by the Nationwide Association of Fostering Providers (NAFP) as *Looking After Yourself, Helping Each Other.*[1] The authors wish to thank ISP, NAFP and especially Andrew Fox and the Teynham carers who made this project possible.

---

[1]   Available at www.johnwhitwell.co.uk/wp-content/uploads/2014/07/Looking-After-Yourself-helping-each-other.pdf

CONTENTS

PREFACE

Dr Andrea Warman was a children's social worker before returning to study for a doctorate in social anthropology. Her research in Havana, Cuba, focused on women's experiences of the Cuban revolution, and shaped her conviction that much can be learned from personal stories and accounts of everyday life.

She has taken this perspective to her projects with foster carers over the past ten years, and written about the meaning of shopping, cooking and eating together in fostering households in the UK and internationally.[1] More recent work for the Nationwide Association of Fostering Providers (NAFP) looked at the creative strategies carers use to prepare young people for adulthood,[2] but raised her concerns about how the challenges and responsibilities of fostering impact on health and wellbeing. At the same time, as a member of the team who piloted the new Adoption Support Fund, she had taken part in discussions with adoptive parents who were also feeling the strain and looking for help.

So she was delighted when NAFP and ISP, an independent fostering agency, gave her an opportunity to try a very different approach to supporting carers, and a chance to work in partnership with Liz Lark. Liz is an experienced yoga teacher, retreat leader and artist. She has authored a number of publications and made *Yogalibre*, a DVD.[3] Over the years her yoga clients have included Alan Rickman and other high-profile actors, dancers and the Monteverdi Choir led by Sir John Eliot Gardiner, but

---

1   Warman, A. (2009) *Recipes for Fostering*. London: British Association for Adoption and Fostering.

2   'Staying Put and Moving On', see www.nafp.co.uk/staying-put-and-moving

3   For a full list of publications and more information about the DVD, see www.lizlark.com

she is passionate about bringing yoga into people's lives, and has a great interest and respect for what carers do. Liz had met Andrea on one of her retreats, and together they developed a programme that would introduce the breathing techniques, *asanas* (poses) and mindfulness meditation to a group of foster carers over a number of weeks.

They were then very fortunate to collaborate with Andrew Fox, who manages ISP's centre in Teynham, Kent. Andrew firmly believes that valuing foster carers and providing excellent support is key to carer retention, and he has held fortnightly lunchtime meetings where carers can talk and help each other at his centre for some time. Andrew is always keen to develop practice, and he was prepared to take a risk and run the pilot programme as an extension of the lunchtime meetings. His staff, especially Rose Mason, also came on board, and their enthusiasm and commitment helped to make this project such a success.

Liz had already worked with Alli Godbold, and she agreed to contribute to the pilot by running a session on good nutrition, encouraging the group to put her ideas into practice by cooking some of her recipes[4] together. Alli began her career as a fashion model, when travelling the world created an interest in making food that is both exciting *and* does you good. Back in the UK she qualified as a nutritional therapist, setting up a practice within a chain of health clubs as well as working alongside local doctors and for The Food Doctor™. Alli currently manages her own practice, offers consultations and runs cookery workshops from her home in London. She also enjoys working in the community, teaching healthy cooking and eating to children and families with disabilities through the Adventures in Eating project.

Together this team ran the programme in Teynham. Yet it would never have been possible without the carers who were willing to go with it. There was a core group of ten: Carole, Marie, Ray, Theresa, Barbara, Jenny, Debbie, Jake, Linda and Patrick. They have been fostering for different lengths of time, and have a range of different experiences in this role, but they are all currently looking after some of the most challenging young people – and share a passion for what they do.

---

4   Some links to Alli's recipes are featured in Chapter 5, and more can be found in her
     publication, *Feed Your Health*; see also www.feedyourhealth.co.uk

Andrea evaluated the impact of this new approach to carer support,[5] and there were positive outcomes – not least the sense of community that this experience encouraged, and how those who took part welcomed this. And the team are so pleased that their approach can now be shared through this book. The additional ideas, tips and stories presented throughout come from the Teynham foster carers, with some input from other carers and adoptive parents Andrea has met and worked with over the years.

The exercises and practices in Chapter 8 are from Liz's earlier work with children, and photographs in that chapter are from her book.[6] The rest of the photography comes from the Teynham pilot, taken by Scott Wishart,[7] that he and the carers have generously allowed to be used here.

Andrea, Liz and Alli went on to do more limited work with a small group of young women in foster care, running a cookery workshop and a short series of sessions introducing basic yoga and breathing practices. Material from these sessions appears in Chapter 9.

The team remain very keen to spread the word, and they know that there are many more foster carers, adopters and their families who would feel the benefit – and should be encouraged to try a different way…

---

5   NAFP (2014) *Looking After Yourself, Helping Each Other*. Available at www.johnwhitwell. co.uk/wp-content/uploads/2014/07/Looking-After-Yourself-helping-each-other.pdf

6   Lark, L. (2010) *Yoga for Kids*. London: Carlton Books Ltd.

7   See www.wishart.photography

● ● ● CHAPTER 1

INTRODUCTION

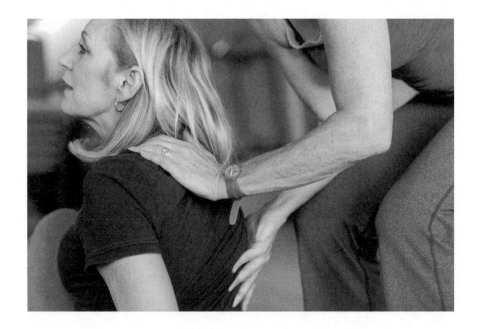

'The root of compassion is compassion for oneself.'[1]

Looking after our health should be a priority for us all – and even more so when we have responsibility for other people. If we don't care about ourselves, how will we find the energy and *vitality* needed to care for others?

---

1   Pema Chodrun, Buddhist monk.

What is 'vitality'?

Vitality has a number of uses and meanings that broadly relate to our health and wellbeing. As a noun, it is often used to refer to the body's *vital* organs – those we depend on for good physical health. When these organs are functioning properly and working together to maintain balance, we have energy and feel healthy and well.

But when describing ourselves or other people as feeling *vital*, we are usually referring to more than this. It's a sense of essential aliveness – being vivacious, animated, having high spirits. Or even having a sense of purpose, focus and meaning – enjoying what we are doing and knowing that it counts.

So finding and maintaining our own *vitality* depends on more than simply keeping physically fit. We need to be aware of our mental and emotional health too, and find ways to nourish and look after ourselves. And this isn't always as easy as it sounds in a world where things change so quickly, where there are many stresses, and where we are under pressure to keep moving – with few opportunities to step back and reflect. It shouldn't be surprising, then, that as we get older we can find ourselves feeling tired all the time, or low and depressed – even losing our sense of self and the person we used to be.

Why is maintaining vitality so important for carers?

Although caring for others may be rewarding, no matter how much we love or value those we look after, being a carer is far from easy. Whether we are a parent, have responsibility for an older family member or for an adult with disabilities, it can be hard to find the time to continue doing the things we enjoy and that make us happy. Being irritated and resenting those who rely on us are natural responses in these situations, and without the right support, even our capacity to empathise can be undermined – especially when there is no respite and we begin to feel under-valued.

Foster carers and adoptive parents are especially at risk, and the complexity of these roles is at last being acknowledged. Yet, in the fostering world at least, expectations continue to grow. The introduction of policies and practice that *increase* foster carers' responsibilities in education, health and safeguarding may be welcomed by some, but they have not always been accompanied by the required support. And it's sadly evident that too many adoptive parents have been left to manage on their own – not knowing who they can ask for help, and not always receiving the help they need when they ask.

While all caring clearly takes its toll, the essence of what foster carers and adoptive parents *do* means that maintaining and 'topping up' energy and vitality is absolutely necessary to keep doing it well:

- Foster carers have always looked after children who have complicated histories and who may have lived in a number of homes and families. This is now often true for adopters too. Understanding these journeys requires effort for the children and young people, but it can also have an impact on the adults who try to help them make sense of their past, and who they are.

- Bringing up children who have been in the care system also involves encountering some degree of loss – at the very least the child's lost opportunity to grow up with their birth family. But foster carers in particular have to learn to cope with multiple losses. Children will move on – sometimes to be adopted, or maybe to go back home. This can be painful enough. There are also not always happy endings, and it can be very stressful when you feel anxious about what the future might hold for a child who could not settle with you and is going to another placement, or a young person who must now leave care before you feel they are ready.

- This all takes place in your own home. Carers may be part of a team who have shared responsibilities for a child or young person. But contact between a birth family member and the child may happen in their living room, or they may have to host other meetings there. Carers don't leave work at the end of the day – they are always on 'duty'. The boundaries between their personal and professional life are by necessity blurred, and they are required to accept a level of scrutiny over how they live that most people would struggle with.

Sharing your home, sharing your life

The emotional impact on foster carers and adopters may be even more intense because they are usually looking after children and young people from troubled backgrounds, and in particular circumstances. The Teynham project provided some valuable insight into the participating foster carers' day-to-day experiences and the feedback we received was that sharing their homes with very challenging young people could even impact on their own sense of self.

Living with someone who has no understanding of their emotions

All of the Teynham foster carers were looking after older children and young people who had chaotic, often abusive early lives, and who had been placed with a number of families since coming into care. While their training and preparation had provided knowledge about why this might create ongoing problems, it could still make that child very hard to live with.

And it wasn't necessarily angry outbursts or aggression that were most distressing. Sometimes it could be sharing a home with someone who was very low or withdrawn. Or with someone who regularly self-harmed. Or, as this carer described, a young man whose unpredictability and mood swings were disturbing her own sense of wellbeing.

> 'If you can imagine. It's like a roller-coaster... There'll be days of calm. Then extreme behaviour. And you don't know why. What provoked that outburst? Because he doesn't know himself. And there are some terrible things he has done. Been cruel to animals. Done things I can't even bear to think about... But there seems to be no remorse. And that can be so draining...'

Living with someone who cannot trust

The same foster carer believed that looking after her young person was particularly wearing because even over time they had been unable to establish a 'connection'.

'It would be easier if there could be some touch, some way to comfort. But although it's been 20 months that trust is not there. He is just not comfortable being touched. And there can't be any hugs... So when you don't get a response it's really hard to keep positive yourself. You have to make a lot of effort to keep responding in a way that should come naturally, the way it's normal to respond to a person you care about.'

Living with someone when there is no relationship

In this context, building a relationship can be an ongoing challenge.

'You know you didn't go into this expecting to get rewards but you can't help it, it's always good to get something back... And when you don't, all you have in the end is yourself. But sad to say some children will tap into that. And although you know they can't help it, you end up feeling that nothing you do is enough. You can give and give until you just have nothing left...'

Living with someone who doesn't respect you

Carers in these situations and in the middle of complex processes and systems may also be living with children or young people who show them little courtesy, or even respect.

'Whenever he'd come back from contact it would get worse. Stealing from us, refusing to go to bed. We knew his birth father played a lot of games, setting the children against each other. Very nasty stuff. But he would come and bring it all back here. We'd have to pick up the pieces... Then, they'd be telling him, they're nothing. Those carers are nothing to you, and you don't have to do anything they say... The final straw was seeing him being rude to my wife. Doing it in front of our daughter, in front of me. Trying to provoke... It made me feel useless. Worthless. It was all too much...'

Living with someone it's difficult to like

These foster carers were also open about how they struggled with their own feelings in response to some behaviours or attitudes of the young people they were looking after.

> 'For me it's the lies. And it's so extreme that it becomes repulsive. I can see how it can make people turn away. So she says sorry, but then she does it again. So then you ask yourself. What does sorry mean? What does it mean to her? And I'm not saying I don't know why she does it. I'm not blaming her. She's had a horrible time. But believe me, it takes a lot out of you, a lot of effort not to start disliking her like other people do.'

Living with someone who doesn't want to be there

Perhaps most dispiriting of all can be sharing your life with someone who really wants to be with other people – *who just doesn't want to live with you.* The carers felt that this could be a real issue when the children or young people had not been able to understand or accept why they had been taken from their birth parents, and why they could not return to them.

> 'Before the girls came to me they'd been with a long-term foster carer but that broke down because the eldest just kept running away. Running back home to her mum and dad – even though they'd had a bad time there and they'd been taken into care... But the family have their own story... And of course the girls love them, and only want to hear the best. They're both bright, funny girls who are a joy to be with. But I know they just want to go back. No matter how much we do, or put in. Or how much we care... And that can hurt. Of course it does.'

Hearing such detailed accounts from the Teynham foster carers about the many layered emotions that they and their families can experience, it's clear that effective support is needed to promote their resilience and to maintain their vitality. But there is an additional aspect of foster carers' and adoptive parents' role that we believe makes effective support *essential*.

Foster carers and adopters have been given the responsibility of bringing up children who could not grow up with their birth families. So whether or not they hold full legal parental rights, they will always play a key part in teaching life skills and preparing the children for adulthood. Therefore, the way parents and carers live their lives – including how they manage their own health and wellbeing – sets a very important example.

And furthermore, there is potential for good carers to influence and shape the emotional development of the children and young people they are bringing up. Even young people who have joined the household in later childhood can learn from them how to cope with their emotions and self-care. But this takes skill and effort, and it's unlikely to happen when carers lack energy or feel discontented. So investing in looking after our carers, offering a range of strategies that help them look after themselves – *and* encouraging them to pass on their knowledge – is more important than ever.

How will this book help?

'We must free ourselves from the hope that the sea will ever
rest. We must learn to sail in the high winds...'[2]

It would be a mistake to believe that we could ever completely remove the pressures involved in being a carer. They come with the package. And if we spend any time with foster carers and adopters we'll hear about the many rewards and benefits too – not least the moments when they can feel and see how they've made a difference. But if we want carers to be able to keep making that difference (and not at a cost to themselves or their families), we must think more creatively about the kind of support made available.

Most fostering agencies now provide some form of counselling – for individuals, or for the whole family. There may even be a psychologist or therapist as part of the team. Adoptive families are now also more likely to have access to this help too. In both situations there are usually support

---

2   Sailor's quote.

groups available. Some facilitated, some more social, but with the shared aim of providing opportunities to meet others in the same situation, to share experiences and ideas.

There's no doubt that this provision can help. But 'talking therapies' are not for everyone. We don't all find it easy to open up and discuss our feelings one-to-one or in a group. And some foster carers can spend a great deal of their time already in meetings or situations being asked to describe what's going on. Adopters – who've been through a lengthy approval and 'matching' process – may also feel 'talked out', at least in the short term.

So the ideas we're presenting in this book are different. They involve *doing* and *being* rather than talking. They may be used to compliment other more traditional support. Or for some, they may be a welcome alternative. And rather than attachment theory or other psychological approaches they draw on the principles of *yoga* and *meditation* with accompanying advice about the value of good *nutrition* and eating well.

Why yoga?

Many people associate yoga with alternative lifestyles and mysticism, and dismiss it as not for them. Some men view it as a bit 'girly', and not for them either. And others believe that it's only for the extremely flexible and super-fit.

But yoga really can be taken up at any age, and by people who are not in the best physical condition. In its traditional form yoga is a philosophy of all-round personal development – a gentle way to *good health* in the broadest sense. It has been in existence in different forms for thousands of years, encompassing mind, body, spirit – your attitude to yourself, others and the world around you.

This yoga practice is based on the understanding of a union between body and mind. When both are functioning in harmony, we feel 'balanced', relaxed, calm and have a sense of wellbeing. However, when we experience too much stress, this can lead to imbalance and, over time, physical, mental and emotional difficulties. Practising breathing techniques, stretches, *asanas* (postures) and relaxation aims to restore and maintain equilibrium, with a number of proven additional health benefits:

- physical flexibility and strength

- increased energy

- improved digestion

- improved posture

- improved sleeping patterns, and ability to rest

- improved ability to relax and reduce anxiety

- lifted mood.[3]

But perhaps even more importantly in this context we believe that yoga is not just a system of physical exercise or a means of switching off from our routines. Rather, it can provide a means for us to *explore* the mind and body, to connect with ourselves – and so promote reflection and change. Then it becomes something we can use to reduce and handle stress – encouraging us to become more centred, and so better able to cope with challenges. It may also help with the development of confidence and self-esteem, especially through learning to coordinate breath and movement. Through *mindfulness* practice, self-awareness may increase, helping us to *respond* rather than *react* to difficult situations. And it has the potential to nourish, replenish and even encourage the development of our vitality – providing the energy we may need to keep going.[4]

So a very good case can be made for introducing yoga to foster carers and adopters as a potential coping strategy, especially if we acknowledge the everyday stresses, increasing pressures and emotional content of their everyday lives. And it may also provide a much needed tool for carers, a

---

3   For further information about yoga, and a discussion about the benefits to health of regular practice, see Lark, L. (2001) *Yoga for Life*. London: Carlton Books Ltd; see also Lark, L. and Goullet, T. (2005) *Healing Yoga*. London: Carlton Books Ltd.

4   For more discussion about the broader benefits of yoga, see Lark, L. (2008) *1001 Pearls of Yoga Wisdom: Take Your Practice Beyond the Mat*. San Francisco, CA: Chronicle Books.

way to pass on these key life skills to the children and the young people they look after.

Why attention to nutrition?

'Eat foods that are tasty, wholesome and satisfying, that give long life, vitality, strength, health, happiness and satisfaction.'[5]

People who are very serious about yoga practice believe that it's as important to care for the inside of the body as it is to keep physically strong and fit. As a result, they pay attention to what they eat and drink to ensure that their digestive and other systems function as they should.

But there are other very good reasons why foster carers and adopters should try to eat well. As we've described, these roles require energy. Carers can be left short of time, so it's tempting to eat takeaway meals or convenience foods. These may provide a short-term boost, but there is plenty of evidence about the long-term damage they can do.

And if we rely too much on these products we can forget the pleasures of enjoying seasonal fruits and vegetables – especially the satisfaction of making a meal from ingredients that perhaps we or our friends have grown.

We can also forget the social value of cooking and eating together. Sitting around a table in the morning or evening with those we live with provides valuable moments to catch up, share stories from the day and to wind down. And making even a simple dinner can be enjoyable and a chance to be creative, especially if it involves working together.

We also need to remember that many of the children and young people who are in foster care or who have been adopted have not had these positive experiences with their birth families. Introducing them to the joys and fun of cooking and eating together are as are important as teaching the practicalities and skills of cooking and budgeting needed for adulthood.

So throughout this book you will find tips and suggestions to encourage carers and their families to eat healthily. And there is a whole chapter

---

5   Bhagavad Gita (400–300 BCE).

(Chapter 5) contributed by Alli Godbold, a qualified nutritionist, describing the changes we can all make to improve our diet, with some of the recipes she has already shared with the foster carers as part of the Teynham project – showing how easy it is to put her ideas into practice.

Tried and tested

Most important, everything presented here has either been contributed by an adopter or foster carer through Andrea's long career in this area of work, or it has been introduced by Liz, Alli and Andrea to carers during the Teynham project – with the impact evaluated. So, we would like to suggest the following:

- If you are working for an *adoption* or *fostering agency* we would like you to consider our ideas and how they might add value to what you do. The structure of this book is based on our pilots with carers, and could provide the outline for a programme you might introduce.

- If you are a *professional* involved in providing support, we'd like you to review your approach following our suggestions and think about how they might be applied to the carers you work with.

- If you are a *foster carer* or an *adopter*, we want to *inspire* you to make the change. We think that you, like Carole, one of the Teynham carers, will *feel* the difference:

'Yes I've lost weight. I'm moving differently. Lighter... But it's more than that. I can't really put my finger on it. All I know is that I've just calmed down and chilled out. Overall just feeling better in myself despite everything that's still going on around me...'

CHAPTER 2

MAKING THE CHANGE

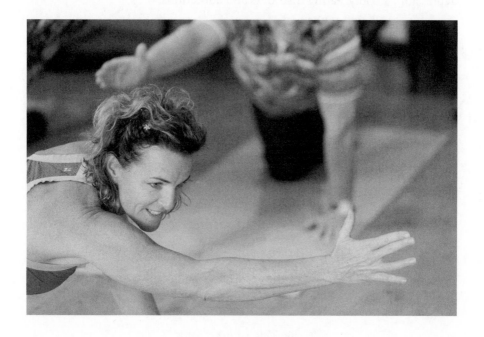

'Begin where you are.'[1]

Making any changes to our lifestyle can feel daunting, so be kind to yourself and take small steps. In time, the breathing and yoga practices we'll show you will help enhance your mood and wellbeing. But simply paying more

---

1   Viniyoga.

attention to what is happening in our body, mind and emotions is where it all begins.

Becoming 'mindful'
What is mindfulness?

Mindfulness meditation has its origins in Buddhist practices that are over 2500 years old. Since then, the techniques have been used widely and therapeutically to manage chronic medical conditions, and even to treat depression, anxiety, eating disorders and addictions.

How to begin

1. As you go about your daily tasks, notice what is happening in your *body*. *What* is the sensation? *Where* is it located?

2. At the same time notice the *emotions* that arise. *What* is it I'm feeling? *How* do I recognise I'm feeling that way?

3. Notice *what* is happening, rather than *why*.

4. Ask yourself, what *thoughts* are arising? What am I telling myself about my experiences?

5. Become more aware of your *senses* – sight, sound, touch and smell – and use them to notice *what* is around you, and *how* it makes you feel.

'Feeling light within, I walk.'[2]

Introduce a new way to start your day

- Even before you get out of bed, cradle yourself in the sound that yogis believe brought the universe into being by chanting '*Om*' (pronounced 'aum'). The vibration this sound creates will help you

---

2   This is a Native American prayer, a Navajo Night Chant.

make connections between your body and your state of mind. Take a deep breath in. As you exhale with an open mouth, let the sound 'aaa' well up from deep in your belly. Round your lips to make the sound 'uuu'. Then close your lips to finish with a soft 'mmm'. Repeat the chant until you feel awake and alive.

- Cultivate your awareness when you wake by spending a minute scanning your body, and checking how you feel this morning. Open your mind to what today will bring.

- Simply stretch. As soon as you open your eyes, stretch your limbs like a starfish to get the energy flowing for the day ahead.

- Think positive. A *sankalpa* (dedication) is a phrase in the present tense to fix your mind on positive action. Say to yourself in the morning, 'I feel well. There are many good things in my life. I am ready for whatever the day brings.'

- To create a feeling of inner spaciousness and abundance that will last, make the *Pushpaputa Mudra*, a symbolic gesture that translates as 'handful of flowers'. Kneel and place the backs of your hands on your thighs or knees, fingers pointing diagonally toward each other. Let each palm form an open cup shape, resting your thumbs against your index fingers. Close your eyes and imagine your hands are filled with the most beautiful flowers with fragrant scents and bold colours.

- Wake up in the shower! Stretching your arms overhead in a full-body extension will enhance your awareness, and encourage your vitality. Using a fresh smelling soap or shower gel – especially one that uses natural products like citrus oils or mint – will wake up your senses too.

- Have a bright-coloured breakfast. Enjoy at least three vibrant-coloured foods at your first meal of the day, such as melon, berries and kiwi fruit to stimulate your appetite and your taste buds.

In time, you will become more tuned in, and you can try some of these mindful practices, depending on your mood.

● ●
●
FOCUS ON THE FACE
●

1. Begin to build awareness of your body by doing this simple exercise when it's quiet and you are on your own. You can sit up, or lie down – however you feel most comfortable.

2. Close your eyes and bring your attention to your face. Explore its boundaries. Notice where it begins and ends.

3. Now begin to focus your attention on specific parts of your face. In your mind's eye move around the jaw, the chin, the lips, inside the mouth.

4. Now move to the forehead, the temples, the ears.

5. Noticing your breathing, begin to relax. Don't make any particular facial expression or make any changes. Just allow your face to be there, as it is. Regard it with kindness and gentleness. No judgement.

● ●
●
DRINK TEA
●

1. Notice your five senses – sight, touch, taste, smell and sound – as you sit down with your cup of tea. Make a special herbal, mint or fragrant brew. Or pour it into a cup that you especially like. Explore the tea with your senses. Notice the delicacy of the china. Or note the design. Feel the heat of holding it in your hands. Smell the fragrance.

2. Become aware of the movement of bringing the cup to your lips, noticing any physical response...experience the taste.

3.   Whenever your mind moves away or other thoughts intrude, bring yourself back to your body drinking the tea. And the sensations you are feeling.

MIND DETOX

1.   If you are having a bad day, or are a bit low, find a quiet place and close your eyes. Simply observe your mind for 5 minutes or so.

2.   If any thoughts or emotions arise try not to react or fight the feelings. See if you can just allow things to be as they are.

3.   Try to let all of these thoughts wash through you. And let any of the emotions pass through too. You will feel lighter, and brighter.

Or you could try:

- Walk in nature – not to *get* anywhere, but just to observe the sights and sounds around you. Listen to the birds. Notice the changing seasons and how that makes you feel.

- Enjoy pets or other animals. Watch the way they move. Take them for walks with you, or curl up at home, and observe how they like to be stroked.

- Notice the blossom and the flowers. If you can, grow them in your garden, or even in a tub or windowbox. You might enjoy an allotment where you could plant fruit and vegetables too. If none of this is possible, buy yourself a bunch of flowers and put them in a place where you can smell and see them.

- Try to spend some of your time with supportive people – those who lift you and your mood.

Remember: You can do many of these things *with* your partner and your children – and the calmer atmosphere you are creating at home will influence how they feel too.

Beginning to nourish

Making changes to our diet also begins by becoming more aware of *what* and *how* we eat. The busy lives that carers lead means it's all too easy to get used to preparing quick meals, and finishing them in a hurry.

But if we get into the habit of eating fast, we don't really *enjoy* our food – because it's not in our mouth long enough to be aware of the textures and the taste! This is especially true when we eat while doing other activities, like sitting in front of the computer or television. And this can become usual practice for the whole family – losing sight of how good it can be to sit around a table and share our meals together.

Bringing mindfulness to eating by trying this practice helps to develop our body awareness, and it also reminds us about the pleasures of eating:

1. On your own, and in silence if you can, without any other distractions, try eating a piece of fruit or even a piece of good chocolate. Do it slowly, and focus all of your attention on what you are doing.

2. Notice the textures and how this food feels in your mouth. Notice how your body reacts in anticipation of the next bite. And chew. Or if it's chocolate, let a square or small piece melt slowly on your tongue.

3. Pause between mouthfuls and become aware of the tastes, what you are eating and how it makes you feel.

Later on, you may want to try doing this with a snack or a small meal – using fruit or vegetables with a variety of colours and flavours.

Once we take more notice of our everyday diet, we can then think about eating food that nurtures our vitality. Alli's advice in Chapter 5 will say more about how we can do this, but to begin:

*   Think about your first drink of the day, and try a reviving 'yogi' tea (available from health food shops or even supermarkets) or the juice of half a lemon in a mug of hot water instead of your usual tea or coffee.

- Try to avoid the artificial stimulants found in coffee, tea and alcohol. If you struggle with this, just have one cup of coffee or alcoholic drink each day. But make it a good coffee or glass of wine, and really enjoy that treat.

- Eat food that is in season. If you can, go to fruit and vegetable markets and look at what's available. Find out about the different fruit, vegetables and pulses you might see there and how to cook them. Introduce new ingredients, or try new recipes with what you already use.

- Think about growing produce in your garden. There is nothing more satisfying than making a dish using fruit or vegetables you have grown yourself. If space is an issue, even a tub or windowbox can be used to grow herbs like rosemary or mint that you can use in your cooking.

- Introduce different flavours through the use of new herbs and spices from different countries or regions that you haven't tried before.

- Eat more fresh food and try to avoid the processed or convenience options. Begin to *listen to your body*, and notice what makes you feel good – and what gives you the energy you need.

Remember: Gardening, growing fruit and vegetables can be a lot of fun – especially if you do it with others. Start simply with herbs, strawberries or tomatoes – surprise yourself with what you can do.

Your family will also be more likely to make these changes if you do. Again, involve them by doing these things together – working in the garden, going to different shops and markets, trying new tastes and flavours.

Learning to be kind to yourself

Eating well is a key aspect of caring for ourselves. But people who spend their time looking after others can easily forget about their own needs. And we can all be our own most harsh critics – focusing on our faults or mistakes and forgetting the positives. Foster carers and adopters experience so many more comments, even criticism, from others, especially when things don't go to plan. Learning to offer kindness to ourselves is therefore an essential step in the approach we are presenting here.

We know that this can be a difficult shift to make – wishing ourselves well can go against everything we have been taught growing up. And sadly, carers are far more used to hearing about their faults than hearing any praise – this can be a real challenge!

We suggest you begin by using a practice to offer kindness to others by creating a *Circle of Kindness*.

● ●
●
● CIRCLE OF KINDNESS
●

1. Sitting quietly and comfortably, bring to mind someone you care about. This may be a family member, a partner, a child, a friend – or even a much-loved pet.

2. Imagine this person or animal, holding them in your mind's eye, and offer your good wishes and love. As you are doing this, repeat to yourself:

    May you be well,
    May you be happy,
    May you be free from suffering.

3. Then imagine that person or animal is standing next to you, even holding your hand. Repeat these words:

    May we be well,
    May we be happy,
    May we be free from suffering.

4. Then call to mind someone else you care about, and repeat the same words and sequence to yourself.

5. Continue in this way for as long as you wish, adding others to your *Circle of Kindness*.

6. When you have become more used to this practice, you may be more comfortable to include *yourself* in the circle. Go through the same process, and when you are ready, place one hand over your heart. Then repeat the same phrases:

> *May I be well,*
> *May I be happy,*
> *May I be free from suffering.*

In time, you may always want to end the *Circle of Kindness* practice to include yourself in this way. You may also choose to do this as a practice on its own.

Or if this still feels too strange, or you aren't ready, then you could try other ways to begin nurturing yourself, such as having a professional manicure or pedicure. If this isn't possible, take the time to do this for yourself. Exfoliate, massage and nourish your hands or feet with oils or creams. Even better if they smell good…

It may be difficult, but do try to find regular time to be alone. And if you can, spend that time doing something you enjoy. Read a book; listen to music. Have a bath using scented oils. Or just sit in the garden with the flowers and animals, if that's what makes you happy.

Don't feel bad about paying this attention to yourself.

Remember: The root of compassion is compassion for oneself. And if your family see you doing this, you will be helping them to follow your example.

Tuning in to your body

If you are beginning to make these changes, you will feel ready to prepare for yoga. Your next steps may be to introduce mindfulness practice that encourages a deeper level of body awareness. You could try an exercise using *Mountain Pose*.

• • • • • • • • • • • • • • • • • • •

MOUNTAIN POSE

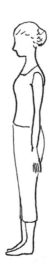

This is a traditional yoga *asana* (posture) that evokes the stillness, strength and innate power of a mountain, grounding the body, but also encouraging uplift in the head – bringing an awareness of posture as well as a positive charge of energy. You can do this at home, but you could also practice when you are standing in a queue, or waiting for a bus or train. Wherever you do it, it is a very good way of practising coming into the body – encouraging your awareness.

1. Stand with your feet parallel and hip-width apart. Feel your toes and heels on the ground.

2. Stretch through the sides of your body upward, keeping your shoulders down and arms relaxed by your side. Imagine a silken thread running from the base of the spine, up through the back of the neck and out through the crown of the head.

3. Picture someone pulling gently on the thread so that there is a small shift, a sense of your head lifting to the sky with your chin relaxing down.

4.   Gaze at a point in front of you. Take a deep breath and relax. Stand tall. Grounded. Connected.

Although the yoga practice we will show you here will be gentle, it's still good to introduce regularly warming up your body at this stage, especially if you haven't been used to physical exercise, or at least not for some time.

These gentle limbering exercises can be done every day on your own in the morning and evening.

• • • • • • • • • • • • • • • • • • •

ANKLE AND WRIST ROTATIONS

1.   Sit comfortably, so you can reach your feet. Then press each of your fingers between your toes, trying to separate and stretch them. Rotate your ankle five times in each direction. Repeat for the other foot.

2.   Make your hands into fists and rotate your wrists five times in each direction. Finish by playing an imaginary piano with your fingers in the air.

• • • • • • • • • • • • • • • • • • •

HEAD AND SHOULDER ROLLS

1.   Sit or stand comfortably and lower your chin down toward your chest. Carefully roll your head to one side – your ear toward your shoulder – and then roll to the other side, feeling your neck muscles ease out. Don't drop your head back. Repeat five times.

2.   Inhaling, lift your shoulders toward your ears. Exhaling, roll them back and down. Repeat five times.

Preparing for yoga

Many people think that they have to join a class to practice yoga, and although there are undoubtedly benefits – having a teacher to guide you as well as sharing your practice with others – it is not essential and you can actually begin in your own home:

- You will need to find a clean, quiet, warm and well-ventilated space, with enough room to stretch your arms to the side and overhead.

- You can practice outside, but again, it should be somewhere quiet where you're away from public gaze and out of direct sun.

- You don't need expensive or special clothes, but you do need to be comfortable. Leggings and a t-shirt are good. Wear things that stretch with your body, and don't inhibit movement. Natural fibres are best.

- Practice with bare feet, but keep some socks to hand to keep your feet warm in the relaxation poses.

- A yoga mat (from a yoga centre, sports shop or online) is a good idea. This will stop you slipping. It doesn't need to be expensive, and can now be bought for as little as £10.

- Some beginners find it more comfortable to use a pillow or folded blanket under their heads or knees when they lie down. You can buy yoga blocks, belts and other props too, later on, but in the early days, you can improvise with books, scarves or cushions.

- Try to establish a time for your practice every day. The ideal times are first thing in the morning (before you eat breakfast) and at twilight.

- It is always best to practice on an empty stomach, so aim to leave at least two hours after eating.

- Avoid practising during the first two days of menstruation. Just relax and meditate. Thereafter, during menstruation do more gentle forward bending, hip opening and restorative poses, and keep your abdomen lower than your heart.

- If you are feeling very stressed or low, it's best to avoid more rigorous yoga. Instead, opt for the gentle poses, breathing exercises and relaxation techniques given in the chapters that follow.

CHAPTER 3

STARTING TO CONNECT

Breathing and Meditation

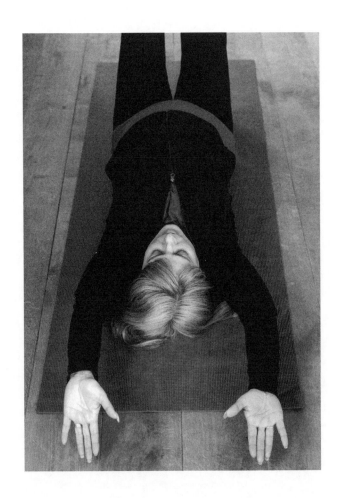

The breathing key (breathing well)

'If you breathe well, you will live long on the earth.'[1]

Yoga is not just about the physical *asanas* (postures). In fact, it is learning and practising a different way to breathe that will probably revitalise you even more than doing the poses.

All too often we become used to taking quick, shallow breaths (into our chest rather than our belly), without making full use of all our breathing muscles, or our full lung capacity. If we carry on with this 'bad' breathing, the result can be physical tension and a whole range of other health problems.

So it's important to become aware of our breath, and return to a natural, deep way of breathing (like we did as a child). This can be both healing and balancing.

The foster carers from our Teynham project told us that they found making this change helped to ground and calm them too, especially in times of stress as Marie explains:

> 'I suppose you get used to shallow breathing and at first I found it hard to slow that down and breathe more deeply. It made me realise how anxious I have been all this time. How tight, how much tension I've been carrying around. But over the weeks I've felt myself relaxing. Accepting things. Letting go...'

You can try doing this exercise, *Three-Part Yogic Breathing*, which encourages full, deep breathing and is the perfect way to start.

● ● ● ● ● ● ● ● ● ● ● ● ● ● ● ● ● ● ● ●

● THREE-PART YOGIC BREATHING
●

1. Lie down with your knees bent up and your feet hip-width apart on the floor. Place a folded blanket beneath your head if that feels comfortable, to encourage your neck to lengthen.

---

1   Indian proverb.

2.   Rest your hands just below your navel. Now observe your breathing for ten full breaths, drawing each deep into your belly. Feel your navel rise each time you inhale, and fall each time you exhale.

3.   Rest your hands on your rib cage and observe your breathing again for ten breaths. As your lungs empty at the end of each exhalation, feel your middle fingers touch. As your lungs fill on each inhalation, feel your fingers separate. At the end of the tenth breath, aim to empty your lungs completely and feel your navel draw toward your spine.

4.   Rest your hands across your collarbones, letting your elbows rest to the sides. As you inhale, feel your chest rise and your collarbones expand towards the side of the room. Become aware of fresh space between your shoulder blades. As you exhale, relax your chest, empty your lungs and feel your navel draw toward your spine.

5.   Finally, practice the first three steps so that you breathe in all three portions of your torso: your belly, your rib cage and your collarbones. This is *Three-Part Yogic Breathing*. Try to keep each inhalation and exhalation of equal length. Follow the flow of the breath, imagining each one as a wave washing through you. Then feel how this steady, calm breathing makes your mind feel like a still, but powerful sea.

Once you have become used to this technique there are other exercises you can use, depending on the time of day, and how you are feeling.

*'Take the breath of a new dawn and make it
part of you. It will give you strength.'*[2]

In the morning, to give you fresh energy, try *Alternate Nostril Breathing*.

---

2   Hopi Nation.

ALTERNATE NOSTRIL BREATHING

1. Sit with your spine straight, resting your hands on your thighs, palms facing upward. Take a few deep breaths to centre yourself.

2. Inhale through both nostrils, then raise your left thumb to block your left nostril.

3. Exhale slowly through your right nostril.

4. Relax your left hand and inhale through both nostrils, then raise your right thumb to block your right nostril.

5. Exhale slowly through your left nostril.

6. Relax your right hand and inhale through both nostrils.

7. Repeat up to 12 breaths (six on each side), aiming to lengthen each exhalation until it becomes twice the length of the inhalation.

When you are facing something daunting and need to boost your confidence, the following exercise, *Balancing Breath*, divides your inhalation into three parts, enhancing your sense of self by slowly filling your body with fresh *prana* (life force).

BALANCING BREATH

1. Sit with your spine upright, bringing your focus to your tailbone. Inhale the first third of breath from your tailbone to the top of your pelvis, then hold.

2. In the second phase of breath, try to feel your breath moving from the top of your pelvis to the space behind your heart, and hold.

3. On the third part of the inhalation, try to sense your breath moving from your heart to the crown of your head, and hold.

4. Exhale, releasing the breath in a wave from the crown of your head to your tailbone.

5. Repeat three times.

Remember: Never hold your breath if you feel discomfort at any time.

If you are having a hard day and feel tired or overwhelmed, this technique, *Skull-Shining Breath*, will spring clean your head, refreshing your brain with energy, leaving you feeling vibrant.

• • • • • • • • • • • • • • • • • • • •
•
SKULL-SHINING BREATH
•

1. Sit with your spine straight and breathe in, expanding your belly.

2. When you exhale, pump your breath out through your nose by forcefully pulling your belly toward your spine.

3. Breathe in, letting the in-breath fill your lungs naturally.

4. Repeat up to 10–12 times.

For winding down in the late evening, *Bee Breath* creates a hypnotic humming sound inside your head, and helps you prepare for sleep.

• • • • • • • • • • • • • • • • • • • •
•
BEE BREATH
•

1. Sit with your spine straight and press your index fingers into your ears to seal off your 'outer' hearing.

2. Close your mouth, separating your teeth and relaxing your jaw.

3. Breathe in slowly through your nose.

4. As you exhale – again through your nose – make a smooth, continuous humming sound.

5. Repeat several times, allowing the sound vibrating inside your head to lull you.

Remember: Changing old habits and making this important shift is not always easy, and you will need to practice. Have patience, because this may take time. Some people can find that singing or chanting are other helpful ways to begin to improve their breathing or to slow down their breath.

We introduced the foster carers in Teynham to a practice inspired by Thich Nhat Hanh, a monk who soothed the distress of people traumatised by the Vietnam War. The Teynham carers found that breathing gently and with mindfulness, repeating these words slowly and silently to themselves, supported their breathing practice. It may help you too:

Ten, I breathe in,
Ten, I breathe out,
Nine, I breathe in,
Nine, I breathe out,
(and so on, counting down from ten to zero)

Breathing, I am here, in this moment,
Breathing, I am happy, in this moment.

Once you are more confident, you can encourage deep and free breathing using these postures – *Fish* and *Crocodile*.

FISH POSE

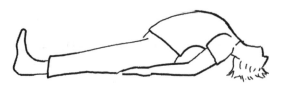

1.   Lie on your back, pressing your pelvis to the floor.

2.   Elevate your chest and head by placing firm cushions behind your neck (make sure your head is slightly higher than the heart). This position facilitates a gentle stretch to the breathing muscles and relaxes the heart.

3.   Breathe slowly. If doing this in a class or with a teacher, they may use a chime bell with this posture that can help you count your breaths, and focus your attention.

CROCODILE POSE

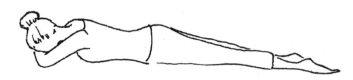

1.   Lie comfortably on the front of your body, face down. Use the palms of your hands to make a pillow stacked under your forehead.

2.   As you inhale, press your navel into the floor.

3.   As you exhale, press your navel back toward your spine. Make a conscious effort to connect with deep abdominal breathing as you continue to do this for the next 5 minutes.

And when you have become comfortable with *Alternate Nostril Breathing*, try this more advanced technique, *Colour Breathing*, which soothes and restores vitality.

● ●
● COLOUR BREATHING
●

1. Sit comfortably with an upright spine. You can do this by sitting with your back against the wall, seated on a cushion if that helps.

2. Close your left nostril with your left thumb and inhale and exhale three times through your right nostril.

3. As you do this, visualise the colour RED, which represents blood flow and the body's circulatory system.

4. Now bring your attention to your spine and breathe up and down the spine three times, visualising the colour MAUVE or PURPLE.

5. Next, close your right nostril with your right thumb and inhale and exhale three times through your left nostril.

6. As you do this, visualise a BLUE/GREY colour, which represents the brain, brain stem and the nervous system.

7. Return your awareness again to your spine, breathing up and down three times once more while visualising the colour MAUVE or PURPLE.

8. Lie down on your back, relax and take several more deep breaths.

'Who looks outside, dreams. Who looks inside, awakens.'[3]

---

3 Carl Jung, 1875–1971.

Doing meditation

Carole, one of the Teynham carers, describes what works for her:

> 'Now when I take the dog for her walk and she's off her lead somewhere quiet, those five or ten minutes they're for me. I do what Liz showed us. Being with myself. Only those few minutes in the day. But it makes such a difference...'

Learning to breathe well is key to practising yoga. The exercises we have suggested here will also help you to focus. And some of the foster carers who used them found that becoming more aware led them very naturally into trying meditation.

Meditation, or *dhyana*, is also a very important part of yoga – especially in your quest to think more clearly, and relaxing more deeply. Regular practice brings about a state of mind fully in the present, which allows you to observe what is going on in your body *and* mind without becoming distracted.

There is an exercise that makes a very clear link between awareness of breath and mind. It is also a quick way of shifting gears and coming into the present moment. The *Breathing Space* encourages us to pause and go from 'doing' mode into 'being'. It helps us to notice physical sensations, thoughts and emotions – while also tuning in to our breath. So it's a kind of 'mini-meditation' – only taking a short time, and possible to do anywhere – which can be used at moments of difficulty, or can become a regular part of our day (as for Carole above). In fact, it can easily be practised while travelling on a train or bus. It's also a very good introduction to meditation techniques.

● ●

● BREATHING SPACE

● You can be sitting, standing, or lying down, and no one will need to know you are doing this.

　1.　Acknowledge what you are thinking, what physical sensations are in the body, any emotions you are feeling. You are *noticing* and *naming.* Try to avoid the tendency to analyse or judge what you notice. Just acknowledge what, if anything, is there.

2. Bring your attention to your breath, and begin feeling the sensations of breathing. It can be helpful to repeat the actions to yourself (or you can repeat the words of the breathing exercise we introduced earlier).

3. Next, widen the focus of your attention from your breath to include the whole body. Become aware of how your feet are rooted on the floor, or your buttocks in contact with the chair if you are seated. Become aware of the room or space you are in. What are the sounds, what are the smells?

4. In this alert state of awareness, you will be in the present moment, free from the thinking mind's whirring and ready for your day.

When you first try this, you may find that your mind will keep darting from thought to thought, or emotion to emotion. But if you keep practising – watching yourself and gently clearing your mind – you will find more clarity and be calmer.

And the more you do it – and as time goes on – it will become easier to reach an awareness of simply *being*.

You may now want to move on from this particular exercise, and try other ways to practice, but it's important to know more about the basics before exploring the techniques any further.

Preparing to meditate

Make a time for your practice each day – the best time is on rising in the morning, or before going to bed. But it's more important that it's time you make for yourself which fits with your routine. If you only have your dog-walking time then that's a good enough beginning!

Begin with 10–15 minutes' daily practice, and try to build up gradually.

Try to find a clean, quiet, well-ventilated room where you feel comfortable. Wear warm, loose clothing, and place a blanket or rug underneath you.

If you find the practice makes you fall asleep, have a refreshing shower before you begin to help you keep your focus.

Meditative sitting postures

Try using these key postures:

● ● ● ● ● ● ● ● ● ● ● ● ● ● ● ● ● ● ● ●
● EASY POSE
●

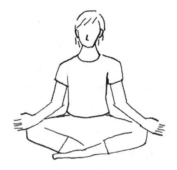

This is the traditional meditation pose. If you feel any discomfort when doing this, sit on a cushion, yoga block or folded blanket.

1.　Sit cross-legged on the bony part of your buttocks and lift your spine as straight as possible. Place your hands on your knees, palms facing upwards.

2.　Close your eyes and relax your whole body, while maintaining alertness in your spine.

THUNDERBOLT POSE

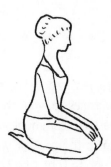

Thunderbolt refers to the energy channel that links the nerve pathways to the brain, encouraging spiritual awareness. This pose is good for meditation because it keeps the spine and energy channel alert and awake.

1. Kneel with your knees together, a cushion, yoga block or folded blanket beneath your sitting bones if you wish. Anchor your sitting bones well.

2. Stretch the front of your ankles and toes, and point your heels up. Rest your palms on your thighs. Close your eyes and maintain alertness.

Once you are more experienced, you can begin to develop your meditation practice and try some of these ideas to find what works for you. You may like to introduce *visualisation* – building on the *Colour Breathing* we've shown you, using your imagination to encourage focus, and even shift your mood.

MOONLIGHT MEDITATION

When too much is going on, and you feel your inner balance is disturbed, sit upright in your meditation posture, close your eyes and imagine your mind as a still lake at night. Picture your thoughts as ripples gently moving across the surface of this calm, moonlit lake. When a thought lingers as more than a ripple, disturbing the still water, focus on the moonbeam lighting it up and trace your awareness back to its light-source, the mystical moon. Allow its soothing glow to seep in to your being, bringing a deep sense of calm.

● ●

THROAT MEDITATION

If your relationships are strained, lie down comfortably on your back, close your eyes and take your awareness to your throat, which, in yogic thought, symbolises purity and heartfelt communication. Consciously relax your throat: imagine it dropping to the back of your neck, open, unrestricted and spacious. Visualise turquoise light (the colour associated with throat *chakra*, or energy) bathing it, and bringing the healing you need to connect with others.

● ●

WAVE MEDITATION

When you've had a hard day and you're having problems winding down, sit upright with your eyes closed and visualise the sea. Watch the waves roll in, and become aware of the release that comes as each wave breaks. Over time, try to exhale as each wave breaks. If you have the opportunity, you can practice doing this sitting facing the sea and watching real waves. Or you may find that using a prop, such as a Tibetan bell, helps you to tune in.

● ●

TIBETAN BELL MEDITATION

To refresh your mind and energise, sit in your meditation posture in a quiet place, where interruptions are unlikely. Buy or borrow an old-fashioned bell that you can chime, and let the sound waves reverberate inside you. Imagine that these chimes are cleansing your ears, nose and eyes – all of your senses. This works best when you are practising with a teacher, or as part of a class as they can take responsibility for chiming the bell, and you can focus on your practice.

LOTUS MEDITATION

Since ancient times yogis have used the rich symbolism of the lotus flower in meditation. But if you prefer, you can buy or pick a single, beautiful fresh flower from your garden, and use it as your focus. Or plant a hyacinth bulb in a small pot in winter and watch it grow. The unexpected colour and scent at this time of year will inspire you.

CANDLE GAZING

To deepen your practice, cleanse your vision and help maintain concentration, sit in a quiet place in your mediation posture about 1m (3ft) in front of a lit candle. Be aware of your straight spine and your breathing. Focus on the flame, gazing intently at it until your eyes just begin to water. Then close your eyes and visualise the flame in your mind's eye for another 2 minutes to develop your inner focus. Now open your eyes a little, becoming aware of a simultaneous inner and outer awareness. Finally, open your eyes fully. Lighting a candle during the dark days of the winter months and noticing the light and warmth of the flame can also lift your mood, especially when you are feeling tired or low.

MANDALA MEDITATION

To nourish your mind, and restore calm when the going gets tough, gaze at a *mandala* for 10–20 minutes. (A *mandala* is a circular pattern traditionally used for meditation and religious devotion, such as a Buddha image.) Allow your eyes to range over its colours and patterns, absorbing the images rather than trying to interpret their meaning. Lose yourself in the magic 'circle' as it guides you towards deeper peace. You can find examples of *mandalas* in yoga or meditation literature. Or try using this one Liz created for the Teynham foster carers, which celebrates yoga rather than any religion or faith:

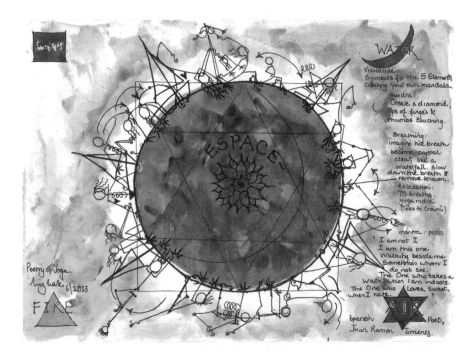

Remember: It can feel strange – and even selfish – to focus this intensely on yourself, especially if you are a carer who is more used to meeting the needs of others. But regular use of the practices we've shown you will encourage mental space, which is essential to keep healthy, and to fully relax, especially if our everyday lives are as stressful as yours can be.

Daily meditation can help us to become more aware of our thoughts and emotions – so we are better able to manage them. Your partner and family will feel the benefit of your more positive mood, and may also be encouraged to try meditation with you. Practising with others at home or in a class can definitely bring its own pleasures. You may find the encouragement and support of a good and inspiring teacher particularly rewarding.

We've found that carers really enjoy doing the breathing, meditation and all of the yoga practice together – so we strongly recommend that agencies provide opportunities for their carers to try our ideas as a group. We'll say more about how you might do this in Chapters 9 and 10, but first we introduce the yoga postures and sequences, exploring the benefits to your health and wellbeing of moving with the breath.

CHAPTER

STANDING TALL

Yoga for Strength and Energy

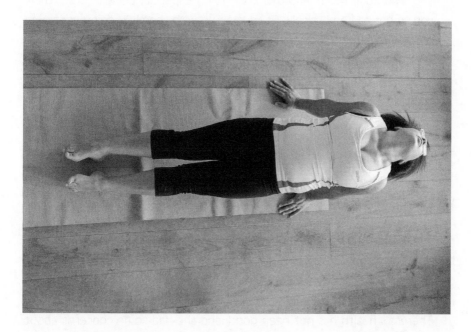

This is the first of three chapters (4, 6 and 7) that introduce the basic *asanas* (postures), balances and some simple *vinyasas* (sequences of linked movements) that you can begin to use in your yoga practice.

We have selected these by drawing on our project work, listening to carers about their needs, and the impact of yoga on their health and wellbeing. Here we present suggestions to support physical strength and good posture along with improvements in energy and focus, which carers told us they valued.

RAY'S STORY ● ● ● ● ● ● ● ● ● ● ● ● ● ● ● ●

Ray is a foster carer in his late forties. He and his wife have been carers for over ten years, and now offer more short-term 'emergency' placements for mainly older children and young people. In this role, there can be a good deal of uncertainty and change.

Ray has always done all kinds of exercise, but was rather wary about trying yoga which he felt might be a bit 'airy fairy.' But he became enthusiastic as a result of the changes he noticed.

'You're getting older aren't you? And if you're sports mad, as I've always been, you do know that you're slowing down, can't keep up like you used to. That can worry you. Because if you don't do as much, then one day you can't do as much. And that is worrying. Especially being a carer. I think you've got to be physically fit to keep up with them! So doing yoga, you know you're doing something. I'll keep on because I just move better. And it's made me notice people older than me who are still flexible. And that makes me want to keep doing it more. I'm getting there, and I want to keep it up.'

THERESA'S STORY ● ● ● ● ● ● ● ● ● ● ● ● ● ●

Theresa is in her mid-fifties and joined her current fostering agency a few years ago – although she had previously been a foster carer for her local authority for over a number of years. She has a 16-year-old son, and for the past year she and her husband have also been looking after a nine-year-old boy, who may continue to live with them long term. However, he had a very difficult early life, has had many disruptions since coming into care, and his behaviour can make him very hard to live with.

Theresa's health has not been good, and she had some concerns about yoga practice.

'I have a bad back and a bad knee, and I did worry about that. But all the stretches really help. And my posture. It's just reminded me to sit better. Then there's the menopause of course...stressing you out in unexpected ways. Physically doing this though makes me feel better. And even my husband has noticed and said, "It's really done you the world of good. You look a different person – please keep on with it!"'

Warming up

Whether you try this at home – building up your own programme or routine – or whether you practice as part of a class, it is always important to prepare for yoga by warming up. We suggest beginning with the warm-ups from Chapter 2, but adding these exercises before the *asanas* (postures) that follow.

● ●

● BREATHE DEEP INTO THE SPINE
●

1.   Lie on your back, semi-supine, which means in a comfortable position with your feet hip-width apart, knees bent and arms by your side.

2.   Place your hands palm down on your navel with the fingers of both hands touching.

3.   Inhale deeply through your nose,[1] and as you do, notice how your navel rises and what happens to your hands.

4.   Exhale through your nose, and notice how your navel falls, and your fingers move closer together.

5.   Repeat for 5–6 breaths.

6.   Then, do the same inhalation, but this time exhale through your mouth, gently releasing the breath. It might help to visualise that you are misting a mirror as you do this.

7.   Repeat for a further 5–6 breaths.

---

1   During yoga practice you are encouraged to breathe in and out through your nose – unless a particular posture or technique instructs you to do otherwise.

• •

ARMS STRETCH THE SPINE

1. Now, in the same semi-supine position, inhale, and as you do, sweep your arms overhead and if you can, rest them on the floor behind you.

2. As you begin to exhale, sweep your arms back down to the sides of your body.

3. Repeat for 5–6 breaths, noticing how your spine relaxes, and how your chest opens through these simple arm movements.

• •

HIP LIMBERS

1. Still lying on your back, inhale, and as you did before, reach your arms overhead, but this time, as you do so, stretch out your legs and extend through your toes.

2. As you exhale, hug your right thigh to your lower belly and squeeze it, almost massaging your lower belly with your thigh.

3. As you inhale, release that leg, reach your arms overhead and stretch out.

4. As you exhale, hug your left thigh into your lower belly.

5. Repeat five times on each side, trying to lengthen the outbreath and so release any tension.

This exercise is called *vatnyasana* (hip limbers), and although it can be used to warm the hamstrings and begin to open the hips, it is also an *asana* known as 'wind-relieving pose', which helps maintain a healthy digestive system by stimulating the internal organs.

You might want to move on from this warm-up routine into an adaptation of the pose that continues this focus on your digestion, and encourages energy flow at the start of any practice.

KNEES-TO-CHEST POSE

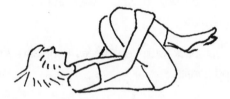

1.   Still lying on your back with your legs out in front, take a deep breath in.

2.   As you exhale, this time hug both knees into your chest, drawing your thighs to your belly to massage your lower belly.

3.   As you inhale, move your thighs away a little.

4.   Repeat for 5–6 breaths, with your thighs moving in and out very subtly, like a concertina.

Perhaps follow with the first of the basic yoga *asanas*, *Bridge Pose*, which you will use regularly in your practice. If you are doing this on your own, without a teacher, take things slowly. The more often you practice these postures, the more confident you will become. But *always* listen to your body, and never do anything that causes any strain, or that makes you uncomfortable.

● ● ● ● ● ● ● ● ● ● ● ● ● ● ● ● ● ● ●
● BRIDGE POSE
●

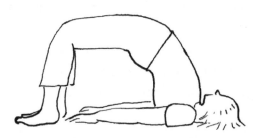

In this pose you will bend into the shape of a bridge, opening up the front of your body, and stretching your spine. It will strengthen your legs, and encourage energy flow to your chest and heart – helping with any respiratory problems.

1.   Lie on your back with your knees bent and your feet hip-width apart and parallel.

2.   Inhale deeply, and as you do, lift your hips and buttocks off the floor so that your body is resting on your shoulders. Your chin should be on your chest. Your arms remain on the floor, stretching toward your heels.

3.   Hold this posture as you take several breaths.

4.   Then lower your back carefully to the floor.

In time, we would encourage you to try *Bridge Flow*, moving in and out of the posture with your breath.

• •
• BRIDGE FLOW
•

1.   As you inhale, lift into *Bridge Pose.*

2.   As soon as you begin to exhale, lower your back as before.

3.   Repeat 5–10 times, trying to slow down your breath, and trying to lower your back, vertebrae by vertebrae, if you can.

4.   You will find that you will lift a little higher each time, and if you are comfortable, try to hold the posture on your final repetition for several breaths.

You may now feel ready to come up from the floor, and try some of the more active, strengthening postures.

• •
• DOWNWARD FACING DOG
•

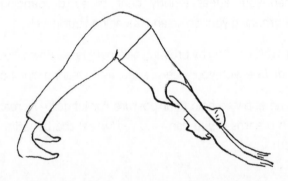

Downward Facing Dog requires you to look downward with your face, resembling a dog stretching. This *asana* is good for circulation as it stretches the whole body. It also helps to build strength in the arms and legs, and boosts energy.

1. Kneel on all fours, with hands and knees shoulder and hip-width apart.

2. Shuffle your hands forward and spread your fingers wide, pressing them to the ground.

3. Inhale, dip your spine, moving the chest forwards, and glide your shoulders away from your ears.

4. Exhale, tuck your toes under, elevate your hips upward, keeping the knees bent at first, so your body looks like a triangle with your hips in the air and your heels on the ground (or raised if you need to).

5. Aim to draw your shoulder blades down your back, releasing your head like a heavy bell to ease tightness from your neck.

6. Take several breaths, anchoring your hands on the mat, and parting your shoulders like curatins across your back.

7. Keep your knees slightly bent to avoid rounding your back, lengthening your spine and engaging your navel.

8. Or *Walk the Dog* by pressing alternate heels down. You can also try *Lady Dog* with your heels raised, as if wearing high heels.

9. In time, try to hold your posture for longer – increasing to up to ten breaths if you can – to really feel the benefits of the brain bath.

• •
• HORSE POSE
•

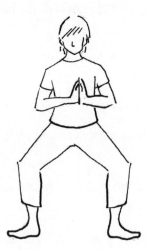

This is a strong, grounding *asana*, named after an animal that was revered in ancient India for its balanced, noble gait. When practised regularly, *Horse Pose* stretches and tones the legs, thighs and buttocks (especially the 'dynamic' variation we describe below). But equally important, it encourages focus and positivity – and so is a very good way to begin the day.

1. Stand with your feet about 1m (3ft) apart (wider than hip-width). Turn your feet out.

2. Bring your hands together at the centre of your chest, as if praying.

3. Bend your knees in line with your toes, aiming in time to take them directly above your ankles.

4. Hold the pose and breathe.

5. This is a stronger posture, and at first you may not be able to hold it for long, so be patient. The more you practice, the easier it will become.

You might want to try *Horse Pose Vinyasa*, where you begin to move in and out of the posture with your breath. It provides more physical exercise, and also brings a flow of energy and openness to the heart area.

● ●

HORSE POSE VINYASA

This is a positive way to prepare for an especially daunting day.

1. Stand in *Horse Pose* with your hands in the prayer gesture, palms together.

2. Inhale, and straighten your legs, raising your hands up through the midline of your body as you do so.

3. Exhale, and circle your arms out to the sides and down towards the floor.

4. Continue this flowing movement for several breaths.

5. Liz also suggests that you try using visualisation with this – as you circle your arms out to the side, imagine that you are scooping up stars in your upturned palms.

6. Then, without stopping, draw your palms together and up through your midline again as you inhale and straighten your legs.

7. Continue for up to ten breaths.

Now with confidence you will be ready to try *Warrior I Pose*, named for its sword-like arm position.

● ● ● ● ● ● ● ● ● ● ● ● ● ● ● ● ● ● ●
● WARRIOR I POSE
●

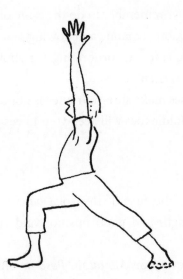

This posture helps to develop physical and mental strength, as holding it requires both balance *and* concentration. Can you be strong and peaceful at the same time?

1. Stand with your feet more than 1m (3ft) apart (wider than hip-width) and with your arms stretched out to the sides at shoulder level.

2. Turn your left foot in a little, and your right foot out by 90 degrees, rotating your legs in line with your feet.

3. Inhale, and lift your chest, stretching your arms above your head.

4. Exhale, and bend your right knee, until it is above your right ankle.

5. Hold for 5–6 breaths, raising your eyes to your hands if you can with a steady, constant gaze.

6. Repeat on the other side.

Warrior I Pose is a strong posture, which again you will find easier over time, and with practice. You can gradually build up the number of breaths you hold for, but always remember to do the same on each side. It can also be easily adapted for more dynamic and flowing practice, and we will show you a *vinyasa*, or sequence, incorporating variations that Liz used with carers at the end of this chapter.

In all *Warrior* poses make sure your knee is not too far over your foot – the knee facing the middle toes will keep your knees protected.

Maintaining focus

Finally, we introduce the first of the yoga *balances*, which support the development of strength and good posture, and cultivate our ability to concentrate.

We've already shown you *Mountain Pose* in Chapter 2 to assist your breathing practice, but this posture is also an excellent way to ground the body – especially if you can hold the stillness it requires. By simply teaching us to stand tall and steady, it helps us maintain a focused mind.

Tree Pose takes us further. Here you emulate the steady balance and vertical focus of a tree, firmly rooted in the earth, yet growing up towards the sun.

TREE POSE

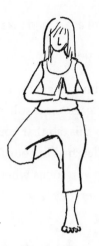

Tree Pose helps with our coordination, and strengthens the legs and spine. It can also help us to keep, or even restore, the attention required to get us through a challenging time.

1. Stand up straight, as in *Mountain Pose* (see Chapter 2).

2. Shift your weight to your left leg, and rest the sole of your right foot on your inner left thigh.

3. If you can't do this (and most people can't when they first try), place the sole of your right foot on your inner calf, below the knee.

4. If this isn't possible, to begin you can simply place your right foot on top of your left, or use the wall to support you.

5. Wherever you are steady, lift your chest, anchor your tailbone and lengthen your spine.

6. Bring your palms together in the prayer gesture. Imagine you have a long root from the base of your spine and the four corners of your feet, anchoring you down in the earth's roots.

7. Hold, and take five deep breaths into the heart.

8.   If you are balanced and you can, stretch your arms above your head, and hold them wide, like the branches of a tree.

9.   Find your steady gaze again, and take a few more deep breaths.

10.   Repeat on the other side.

Tree Pose, like all other standing balances, is not easy when you begin. You will find that fixing your gaze on a still point in front of you helps. Soften your eyes when you do this, so that your gaze becomes meditative and liquid (using what you've learned in your meditation practice). This is called *infinity gaze*. It can help you focus when doing any of your *asanas*, and also with your work and everyday tasks.

● ● ● ● ● ● ● ● ● ● ● ● ● ● ● ● ● ● ●
● EAGLE POSE
●

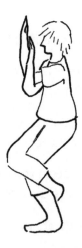

When you are comfortable with *Tree Pose* you can try the more advanced *Eagle Pose*.[2] *Eagle Pose* encourages all-body strength, endurance and enhanced concentration – helping with physical and mental stability.

---

2   If you have any problems with your knees, this is not a good posture for you.

1. Stand in *Mountain Pose*, then bend your knees slightly.

2. Balancing on your left leg, lift your right foot up and cross your right thigh over the left.

3. Hook the top of the foot behind the lower left calf and squat deep.

4. Stretch your arms out in front of you and cross the right arm over the left at the elbows.

5. Raise your forearms with the palms of the hands facing each other.

6. Press the palms together and lift the elbows higher, stretching the fingers upwards, and drawing your shoulder blades down your back.

7. Hold, and take eight breaths. Then unravel your arms and legs and take a breath in *Mountain Pose*.

8. Repeat on the other side.

In your own practice, when you want to boost your inner and outer strength and focus, you may follow our suggestions, or use the *asanas* presented here with other poses from the chapters that follow. You may wish to add meditation or some of the breathing exercises to your routine.

We want to encourage you, or your teacher, to be creative and find what meets your needs. We'd only insist that you warm up first, and then stretch and relax at the end. In Chapter 7 we will show you how to do that.

The carers we worked with enjoyed the *vinyasas*, or sequences of linked poses, Liz introduced, which encouraged awareness of breath – but with a 'lightness' and humour.

So we end this chapter with the *Standing Tall Vinyasa* that gave the Teynham foster carers enough energy, self-confidence and spirit to see them through their week. We hope it will do the same for you.

• • • • • • • • • • • • • • • • • • • •

• THE STANDING TALL VINYASA
•

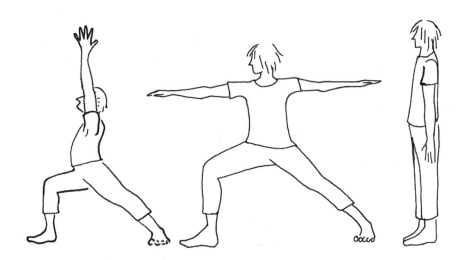

1. Stand with your legs in *Warrior I Pose* with your feet wide apart, your right foot turned out 90 degrees, and your left foot turned inwards 45 degrees (in all *Warrior* poses make sure your knee is not too far over your foot – the knee facing the middle toes will keep your knees protected). Imagine your feet are on two railway tracks, with your navel facing your right knee.

2. Plant the four corners of your feet down, anchoring your big toe joint and the outside edge of your heels. Feel rooted.

3. Lengthen your spine, lift your heart and relax your shoulders down.

4. Inhale, straighten your front (right) leg, and place your hands at your heart, palms together in the prayer gesture.

5. Exhale, and bend your front leg, gliding your knee towards 90 degrees.

6. At the same time (as your exhale and bend your leg) stretch your arms wide open at shoulder level. With your arms held in this position you are in *Warrior II Pose*.

7.   Now repeat the movement five times (straightening your front (right) leg, and placing your hands at your heart on the inhale, and bending your front (right) leg and stretching your arms out on the exhale).

8.   Do this using *Ocean Breathing*, by narrowing the back of your throat – as if gently narrowing a hose pipe – and creating a smooth, hissing sound. This technique encourages more oxygen intake, and flushes out toxins.

9.   Take a short break with two or three regular breaths in *Mountain Pose*.

10.   Return to *Warrior I Pose* on the same (right) side.

11.   With your right knee bent, form two fists with your hands and place the left fist in front of your heart, and stretch your right arm out to the right.

12.   Face forwards, towards your right leg, and take a deep inhale.

13.   Exhale strongly through the nose, and as you do, pump your fists like a boxer – forcing out any stale air.

14.   Remaining steady, take another deep inhale and straighten the front knee.

15.   Exhale strongly through the nose, bending the front knee into *Warrior I Pose*. In this position, pump your fists like a boxer to expel any stale air and frustration.

16.   Repeat this five times to begin (over time you may build up to 10, or even 20 repetitions of the nose and mouth exhalations with arm pumps).

17.   Return to *Mountain Pose*.

18.   Take three deep breaths in this pose, with arm sweeps overhead as you inhale, if you wish.

19. Draw your hands to your heart in the prayer gesture as you exhale, to centre and focus again.

20. Now repeat this *vinyasa* on your left side – this time repeating your dynamic *Warrior I Pose* with *Ocean Breathing* five times over your bent left knee. And then the pumping breath with boxing hands five times looking towards your left leg.

21. To finish, return to Mountain Pose, and after centring, and with legs hip-width apart and knees soft, fold forward from the hips into a Wide-Legged Standing Forward Bend (see *A Vinyasa for Sattwa* in Chapter 6).

22. Take 10–20 deep breaths, hanging like a willow tree.

Now you will feel strong enough for the most challenging of days!

CHAPTER 5

EATING FOR VITALITY

Good Nutrition for Feeling Healthy

The recipes marked with ● can be downloaded in colour and printed out from www.jkp.com/catalogue/book/9781849056649

Becoming 'mindful', learning to breathe well and practising yoga can improve your physical and emotional health. But changing the way you and your family eat is just as important, and there are some very simple steps you can take.

We've worked with nutritional therapist Alli Godbold on our projects, and she has shared her tips and recipes with foster carers and the teenagers they are looking after, showing them that you don't have to spend more time *or* more money, and that cooking and eating together can be even more fun when it does you good:

'I am a nutritional therapist. In simple terms, that means I see clients, explore their health problems and work out a diet plan to help them improve their wellbeing. I have been doing this since qualifying in 1996, and over the years I've come to realise that so many people are really scared of cooking. Or if not scared, they think it takes too much organisation and effort. Especially busy people, short of time who want to be ready and eating within 30 minutes – with minimum fuss…

So that usually means eating a supermarket ready meal, or ordering a takeaway on a Friday night. But I promise you, cooking my way doesn't require tricky skills. It can be easy, satisfying and no big deal. And it will really help you look after yourself. Making your own food is rewarding too. You know what's gone into it, you feel a sense of achievement and it's good for your health – what more could you ask for!'

Alli has compiled a series of ten top tips, things we can do which to improve our energy, balance our mood and help us feel better.

Alli's tips for healthy eating
1. Get the basics right

Eat more:

- Protein – lean meat (like chicken) and fish (especially oily fish, like salmon or mackerel).

- Wholegrains and pulses – all kinds of beans, chickpeas and lentils, even canned, or semi-prepared (you can easily find these now in supermarkets) so that you can save time.

Add plenty of:

- Vegetables and fruit – try not to rely on the same boring vegetables and eat a variety. Green leafy vegetables like spinach, broccoli and kale are especially good for you. And introduce fruit as part of a meal rather than grazing on it throughout the day. Berries can be used to make great breakfasts and delicious puddings.

Introduce:

- Nuts and seeds – you can buy mixtures of these from fruit and vegetable markets, health stores and now from supermarkets. Avoid the salted and roasted varieties that are high in calories – raw mixes are nutritious and just as tasty as a snack, in salads or as toppings.

Cut back on:

- Processed food – ready meals, takeaways, processed meats like sausages, cheese and pizza. They may be what you and your children enjoy, and they may sometimes be the 'easy' option. But they are full of empty calories and contain high levels of salt and sugar that can do a lot of harm.

- Sugary and refined foods – shop-bought cakes, biscuits and sweets. But don't forget the 'hidden' sugars too. Many breakfast cereals (especially the ones that appeal to children) are full of sugar. So are the cans of drink, orange squash and other drinks that are commercially produced. Sugar can also be 'hidden' in ready meals, sauces and supermarket soups. Be careful of eating too much fruit, limit fruit juices to once a day (good at breakfast time) and keep dried fruit to a minimum, as this is a concentrated source of fruit sugar.

Remember: Making any changes to our diet is not easy, especially when we're trying to encourage others to do the same. But you will find it helps if you do this as a whole family. It may be especially hard for older children or teenagers who've come to you with their own tastes and even 'bad' habits. Some may not even have been used to having regular meals. We'll be making more suggestions for what you can do to encourage them in Chapter 8, and ideas for cooking and eating together in Chapter 9. There are children and young people who will come to you with more serious eating issues, and you should always seek help for those. But here we bring you simple ideas from other carers to help you put Alli's tips into practice.

DEBBIE'S TIP ● ● ● ● ● ● ● ● ● ● ● ● ● ● ●

'The first step we took was to begin making the effort to sit down around a table as a family – at least once a day. You can drift in to things like popping something in the microwave for one, something different for another when they come in. Or someone who wants to eat in front of the TV, or when they're on the computer.

But making it more social, more of an occasion – without other distractions – does work. You pay more attention to what you're eating, you notice when you're full. And you might find you enjoy each other's company!

Then you can start thinking about what you're going to eat. Planning it a bit more. Going shopping together. Now we'll sometimes make the effort and go out with the kids to a proper market. They can see what the vegetables look like, choose things they'd like to try. Everyone's part of it then, and it's not just you who seems to be taking things away, or making a lot of boring rules...'

2. Add variety to your diet

We can all get into a routine, or come to rely on the same foods, so try to introduce more variety into the meals you and your family share.

- Try a new fruit, or a new vegetable, every week. This doesn't have to be expensive, especially if you eat seasonally, eating vegetables that are in season and readily available at different times of the year. You might use what you find in your cooking, or you may eat the new fruit at the end of your meal as a healthy pudding. And fresh fruits make breakfast more exciting. Try using berries to make a smoothie in the summer months, or use them as a topping for porridge when the season changes.

  Remember: Fruit can be a winter food. A warm fruit salad with honey is a delicious pudding when it's cold outside.

- Try cooking a new recipe each week too. You'll find plenty of inspiration from television programmes, magazines and online, as well as the more traditional cookery books. You may find family recipes handed down over the years. Or you might ask your friends or neighbours to share their favourites.

Remember: It's good to be curious about food eaten by people from different backgrounds and cultures. You might try cooking Italian, Indian or Chinese food, and add variety by introducing these new tastes and flavours. This doesn't have to be too challenging or take a lot of time. Begin with a soup or a salad that together can make a very satisfying alternative to a sandwich for lunch.

- Notice how your plate looks and aim for a rainbow of colours rather than too much beige. This becomes easier with practice, especially as you begin to try different pulses and vegetables.

  Remember: We eat with all of our senses, and as you are becoming more 'mindful' and aware of what you are eating, having colourful and attractive food will make mealtimes more interesting for everyone.

VERNON AND JENNIFER'S TIP • • • • • • • • • • • •

'We're short-term carers and so we've had to be flexible and be ready to respond to different children and their likes and dislikes. But at the same time make sure they're getting a good meal. All the while avoiding mealtimes becoming a battleground! We're both of Caribbean heritage, but our own boys grew up eating a mixture. They tried all kinds of food, and that's what we still encourage children to do. We might have sweet potatoes as well as rice or bread. Different salads. Plenty of variety, and some choice. Especially in the early days of any placement. So we won't dish up. It's all laid out on the table, it looks good. But the choice is there. And we can get across to a child that you can put on your plate what you're ready to try – what you want to eat.'

3. Know your carbs!

Alli helped our carers to understand that there is a difference between carbohydrates and what they do to our body, our energy levels and our metabolism.

- Opt for the carbs that give a *slow release* of sugar into the system. Vegetables like sweet potatoes, pulses and wholegrains – brown bread, brown rice and wholewheat pasta. They are more satisfying over time, especially if we eat them earlier in the day. So try porridge or oats for breakfast – made tasty and more interesting with different toppings.

  Remember: These new tastes and textures may take some getting used to, so you might want to do this in small steps. Make mash with sweet potato rather than your usual variety. Or make the same bolognaise or tomato sauce as you usually do, but this time serve it with wholewheat pasta. These items are now much more widely available, and you can even buy the same pasta shapes that your family are used to in the wholewheat variety.

- Reduce your intake of refined carbs. It is tempting because if you are tired or flagging these will give you a 'rush', but it's always short-lived. And they will upset your energy balance – contributing to weight gain. So try to cut down on sugary foods like cakes, biscuits and breakfast cereals. And keep your intake of white rice, white pasta and white bread to a minimum.

  Remember: Giving up white bread can be especially tough, along with the shop-bought cakes and biscuits many children and teenagers have become used to. But there is now a great variety of different, healthier breads available. You could even make your own. And we'll be showing you that you don't have to give up eating puddings or cake if you try one of Alli's recipes.

ANDI'S TIP ● ● ● ● ● ● ● ● ● ● ● ● ● ● ● ●

'I've looked after a lot of teenagers over the years and we've held no end of reviews and other meetings in this house. In the early days I wanted to make those meetings (which could be fraught and painful) more welcoming and "homely". So I would make my own fruit cake to share, rather than just open a packet of biscuits. And I always used organic ingredients before it was fashionable to do that. Well the kids would tease me, call it "hippy cake". But I became quite famous for it. And they all remember it. In fact, when some of them come back and visit with their own children, they'll ask for it. So I'm teaching a new generation about this healthy option along with all the memories...'

4. Enjoy your protein!

- It's important to eat plenty of protein, and it doesn't have to be expensive or boring. Alli believes that eggs are an excellent, much over-looked option. They make a great breakfast or lunch. And a tasty Spanish omelette is a real treat for a late morning brunch at the weekend when everyone has more time to sit down together.

- Fish is another good alternative, and the less pricey varieties can be made more delicious if you know how to cook them. Mackerel or salmon coated in seasoned flour and pan-fried, then served with oven-roasted sweet potato wedges, is a healthy (and much cheaper) alternative to fish and chips.

- Chicken can be cooked in so many different ways, and everyone enjoys a good roast with plenty of vegetables for Sunday lunch.

- Nuts and seeds are an easy way to increase your intake as toppings or snacks.

- Don't forget that pulses and beans are an excellent source of protein, and can become the main ingredient in a casserole or a bake, especially if you add plenty of colour and flavour to the dish.

- Or you may become more adventurous and introduce things you and your family have not tried before, like puy lentils, quinoa or tofu.

Remember: Think about how the texture of food can make it more interesting. You might coat a piece of fish or chicken in seeds or crumbs before cooking to make it crunchy. Fresh herbs can be added, or different spices. You might try growing herbs in your garden (or even a windowbox will do). Or you can explore the markets or specialist shops to find out more about diverse tastes as well as the health benefits of eating particular spices like turmeric or ginger.

LINDA'S TIP ● ● ● ● ● ● ● ● ● ● ● ● ● ● ● ● ● ●

'When our little boy came to us his diet was really limited and he would only really eat chicken nuggets, or fish fingers if we were lucky. I didn't push him, or want to make him uncomfortable by giving him meals that were too far away from what he was used to. So I began by taking one of Alli's recipes – and adapting it! So I did coat fish in sesame seeds, but the first few times I used a white fish rather than salmon. And I cut it into fingers. A kind of home-made fish finger – that wasn't too strange. But moving in the right direction...'

5. Don't be afraid of fats!

Not all fat is 'bad' for you. In fact, our bodies need it as part of a balanced diet.

- Oily fish like trout, salmon, sardines or mackerel are a great source (even from tins).

- Nuts and seeds also contain 'good' fats. You might want to try cooking with nut oils, and walnut oil can make for an especially tasty salad dressing.

- Coconut oil is the choice for many different cuisines. It's not expensive, it doesn't make food taste too sweet, and it's a healthy alternative for frying food.

- Try to include avocados in your regular diet. They are an excellent source of healthy fat, and can be used in many different ways. Avocados mashed with lime juice, herbs, and even a little chilli make guacamole, which can be used as a dip with crackers or raw vegetables. Many children and teenagers like it, and it can be a good introduction to this 'super food'. Later you can then try adding avocado to a breakfast smoothie. It works really well with chopped pear and fresh mint, and blends very easily. Once you become more adventurous, chop the avocado with some diced cucumber and a few leaves of baby spinach. Add a couple of dessert spoons of Greek yoghurt, top with a little water and blend. A very healthy start to the day – and one that also tastes good!

Remember: These changes will be easier if you make them together, so take small steps.

6. Become familiar with antioxidants

Antioxidants support your immune system, protect your health and fight degenerative disease, so try to eat food with a high content of them.

- Fresh vegetables and fresh fruit are the best source of antioxidants, and some are especially good for you, so use plenty of green leafy vegetables like spinach, cabbage and kale to make soups, or to accompany your protein in main meals. But don't forget that you can also use them in breakfast smoothies, especially if you buy a more powerful blender. Adding green apple to kale or spinach sweetens the taste naturally, and is very refreshing if you add ice.

- Berries have higher levels of antioxidants than other fruits, so try to eat plenty of blueberries, blackberries, cranberries, raspberries and strawberries. Cherries, plums and some varieties of apple are also good. Eat these as part of your family meals rather than encouraging 'snacking' because they do, like other fruit, contain sugar. They don't have to be expensive if you buy in season, and you might think about trying to grow some of them in your garden.

- If you can, try to drink one or two cups of green tea daily. This will supplement your antioxidants and give a real boost to your immune system – especially when you are under pressure. You could try to make this part of your routine – maybe the first 'mindful' drink of your day, or to relax after your yoga practice. Again, you no longer have to visit a health food shop to buy this product, and most supermarkets stock a range. If it tastes strange, try using a teaspoon of honey to sweeten it, or buy green tea with added lemon for something more familiar.

Remember: It may be more challenging to introduce your family to green tea or curly kale, but even making a simple dessert of fresh strawberries and natural greek yoghurt with honey and mint for flavour will change habits and bring benefits.

CAROLE'S TIP ● ● ● ● ● ● ● ● ● ● ● ● ● ● ● ● ●

'I think all of us remember school dinners and the smell of cabbage cooking which would put any of us off... And some of the teenagers I've looked after have honestly never cooked themselves, and the only vegetables they've tried are frozen peas...

But it's the way you present things isn't it? A bed of buttery, green cabbage with a piece of well-cooked fish on top is so much more appealing, isn't it? And I've found when it's growing in the garden and they see where it comes from, and what you can do with it. Well that makes all the difference.'

7. Find a balance

Sitting down to eat meals with focus and without the distractions of the television or computer will raise your awareness of what and how much you are eating. Alli suggests that we pay more attention to the proportions of food on our plate.

- We should eat a palm-sized portion of protein (fish, lean meat, eggs, tofu, etc.).

- Add a small serving of a starchy carbohydrate (brown rice, brown pasta, sweet potato, etc.).

- Fill the rest of the plate with salad or other vegetables (not potatoes), so that about half of your plate is vegetables.

Eating in this way will help you manage your weight, keep your energy levels stable, help your mood and keep you healthy.

Remember: Children and young people who are still growing and who are more physically active need more of the rice, pasta or other carbohydrates. Trying to control other people's portions is not advisable, but if children see you eating sensibly and in a balanced way, they will learn to do this too.

RAY'S TIP ▶ ● ● ● ● ● ● ● ● ● ● ● ● ● ● ●

'I knew I'd been putting on weight over the years. It just creeps on doesn't it? Being more aware and following Alli's advice made me realise that I was eating when I wasn't hungry. Cutting down on the carbs (especially in the evening) means that I've lost a few pounds – without being hungry! But more than that, I'm feeling less bloated, my digestion's better and I've got more energy. Which is definitely needed when you do what we do.'

8. You don't need stimulants

It can be very tempting when you have a stressful life to keep going by drinking coffee or a can of cola. When time is short you might miss a meal, and have one of these drinks instead. And at the end of the day, when it's hard to switch off, a beer or a glass of wine may be very appealing.

But whether it's coffee, milk chocolate, cola, beer or wine, these are short-term solutions that may lift your mood temporarily, and then cause your sugar levels to crash, leaving you feeling more exhausted. And in the long term, these 'treats' will also play a part in weight gain.

Try to cut right back on these artificial stimulants, and make sure you eat well and regularly to keep your sugar levels stable. This includes diet drinks, which may not have the same number of calories, but still do you harm. In fact, Alli compares drinking these to pouring industrial waste into your system!

You can do this slowly, by replacing your morning coffee with a healthier alternative, and then gradually cutting down over the rest of the day.

If part of your 'treat' is taking a break for your coffee, or meeting with friends or other carers over a coffee or alcoholic drink, try to change this pattern and reward yourself in other ways. You might support each other to make this change. Or taking this time out might become an opportunity to do some breathing or meditation.

But don't be harsh on yourself! You may find it works for you to have one daily cup of coffee, or one glass of wine. So make sure it's good coffee that you can savour, or a good glass of wine that you'll really taste and enjoy.

9. Keep hydrated

Busy people may also forget to drink enough water, and a headache or feeling tired can often be a sign that you have become dehydrated. So get in the habit of drinking water regularly throughout the day.

When you wake, a glass of warm water with a squeeze of lemon or lime is good for your digestion, and a great way to begin the day. Drink water with family meals. Have a jug on the table. Adding ice, slices of fruit and even sprigs of fresh mint, can make it more interesting for everyone.

Tea and coffee can be dehydrating, so if you do have a cup, make sure you also have a glass of water. Always have a drink of water before you go to sleep, and if you can, keep a glass by your bed in case you are thirsty during the night.

Remember: Fruit and herbal teas that don't contain caffeine are a good alternative, especially if you find it difficult to keep drinking water. There is a huge variety to choose from, and you can match your mood and the time of day to your choice. Coconut water (without any added sugar) is a refreshing alternative. It's now on sale in most supermarkets, and is not as expensive as it used to be. Children often really like the taste – and it does them good!

DEBBIE AND JAKE'S TIP ● ● ● ● ● ● ● ● ● ● ● ● ●

'Cutting down on the coffees, drinking water rather than juices or soft drinks was not easy for us. Especially when we came down to our Carer's Centre where the kettle goes on and the coffees start... But we didn't want to avoid going there as that's where we see each other and off-load. Talk and share. So we've done it as a group! Now there's all the different teas to try and we're working through them. At the moment mint for calming is my favourite.'

10. Enjoy your food!

Alli strongly believes that we should enjoy and take pleasure from our food. So a little of what you like is healthy for both the body and the mind. You don't always need to be an 'angel' to feel the benefits.

Follow these principles for 80 per cent of the time, and reward yourself with an occasional 'treat', something that makes you happy. Whether that's a cup of coffee, a slice of cake, a glass of wine or a few squares of chocolate, make it the best you can, and give yourself the time to really make the most of it.

Remember: You are a role model for the children and young people you are bringing up. So if they see you having a healthy relationship with food, it will help their development too.

And now to show you how simple it is to put Alli's ideas into practice, here are four of her recipes, all tried, tested and recommended by the Teynham carers!

First, a soup that is easy to make, packed full of goodness and that makes a satisfying lunch.[1]

---

1   For more of Alli Godbold's delicious recipes, see Godbold, A. (2010) *Feed Your Health: The Nutritionists Guide to Easy, Delicious Home Cooking.* HotHive Books.

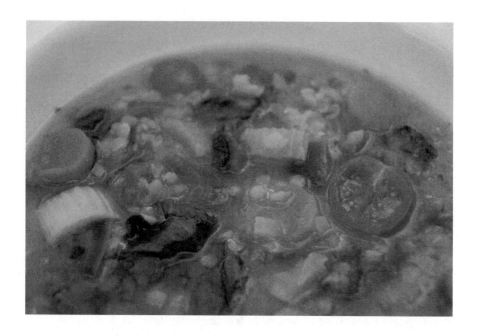

LENTIL AND SPINACH SOUP

Ingredients

2 carrots, peeled and sliced

2 sticks celery, sliced

2 medium onions, peeled and chopped

2 cloves garlic, peeled and sliced

Extra virgin olive oil

Thumb-sized piece of fresh ginger, grated

1 fresh red chilli

10 cherry tomatoes

1.8 litres (1.9 quarts) of stock, using Marigold Bouillon

300g (1½ cups) red lentils

200g (⅞ of a cup) fresh spinach

Sea salt and ground black pepper

Method

Heat a large pan and add 2 tablespoons (⅛ of a cup) of olive oil.

Add the carrots, celery, onions and garlic, and cook for approximately 10 minutes with the lid askew, until the carrots are softened.

Meanwhile, peel and grate the garlic, deseed and slice the chilli finely, and cut the tomatoes in half.

Add the stock to the pan with the lentils, ginger, chilli and tomatoes.

Bring to the boil and then reduce the heat and simmer for approximately 10 minutes with the lid on, until the lentils are cooked.

Add the spinach and let it wilt into the soup.

Serve immediately.

And now, a salad that uses fruit, has texture and flavour, and is far from boring.

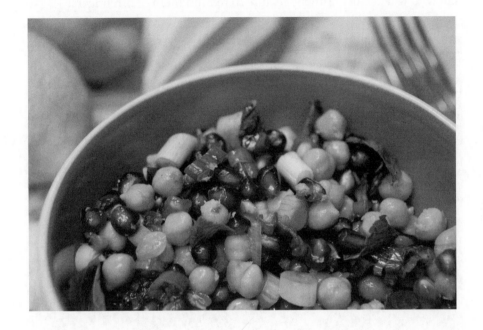

POMEGRANATE AND CHICKPEA SALAD

Ingredients

4 spring onions, finely sliced

1 garlic clove, finely sliced

Small handful of mint leaves, roughly shredded

Olive oil, to taste

1 can chickpeas, rinsed and drained

Grated zest and juice of 1 lemon

2 pomegranates, seeds

Sea salt and ground black pepper

Method

Mix all the ingredients together and season well.

Sesame Salmon is a main course that is based on an oily fish, and is particularly good for children who might be unfamiliar with fresh salmon, but who will like the crunchy texture to remind them of fish fingers!

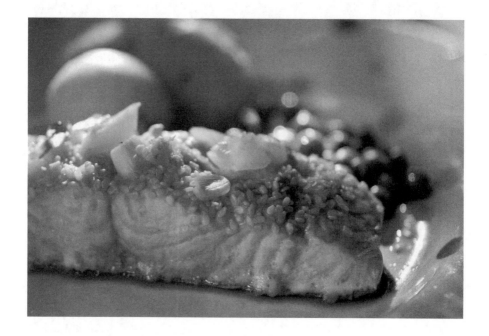

SESAME SALMON

Ingredients	Method
4 salmon fillets, skinless	Preheat the oven to 180°C/350°F.
3 cloves garlic, minced	Place the salmon fillets in an ovenproof dish, cover with rest of ingredients and allow to marinate in the fridge for at least 10 minutes.
Thumbnail-sized piece of fresh ginger, grated	
3 teaspoons sesame seeds	Bake in the centre of the oven for approximately 10 minutes until the fish is cooked through, but not dry.
3 spring onions, sliced	
3 teaspoons tamari soy sauce	
Juice of 1 lemon	

And finally, a zesty pudding to show you that you don't have to give up the things we all enjoy.

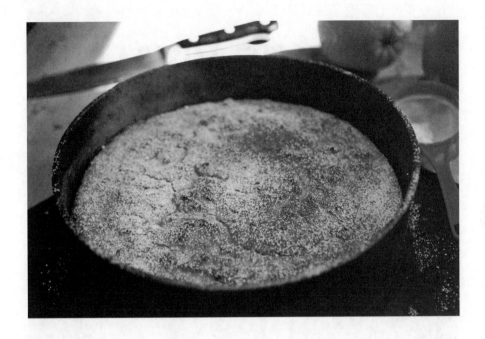

ORANGE TORTE

Ingredients	Method
2 large oranges	Put the whole, unpeeled oranges in a pan and add cold water to cover.
170g (¾ cup) coconut sugar	Bring to the boil, cover and simmer for one hour. Drain and leave the oranges to cool.
200g (1½ cups) ground almonds	Preheat the oven to 180°C/350°F.
4 eggs	Grease a 23cm (9in) round cake tin and line with non-stick baking parchment.
Juice of ½ lemon	
½ tsp baking powder	Cut the oranges into chunks and remove the pips, then tip them into a blender or food processor. Add the remaining ingredients and process until evenly blended, then pour the mixture into the cake tin.
	Bake for 45–60 minutes until risen and firm.
	Turn the torte out on to a wire rack to cool.
	The torte is delicious served warm as a dessert with yoghurt, but is equally good eaten cold.

CHAPTER **6**

RESTORING VITALITY

Yoga for Balance, Calm and Wellbeing

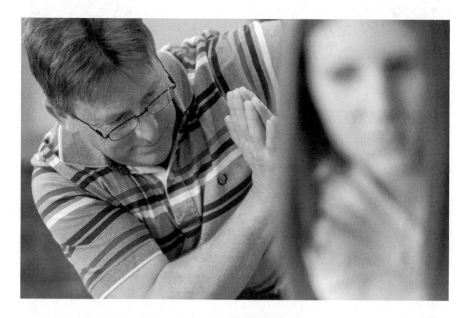

The carers who took part in our projects noticed more than physical changes. Some described feeling calmer, and being better able to cope. So this chapter focuses on the practice we introduced that creates the 'space' needed for reflection, and which may help you to manage your emotions.

CAROLE'S STORY

Carole is a single carer with teenage daughters. She has been fostering a child long term for a number of years, but as this young woman approaches adolescence and is experiencing difficulties at school and understanding her own history, it is becoming more challenging for the whole family.

With travel to therapy and education appointments (as well as the general running around after teenagers), Carole had been finding it hard to make time for herself.

> 'Fostering is 24/7 – seven days a week. It never stops and we don't clock off! So you're always "on". Planning ahead, trying to fit it all in... The yoga's helped me slow down, take a pause. Given me time to think. About what you can do. And what you can't...'

There are *asanas* (postures) that are 'restorative', and that are especially good to use for this purpose. Again, we want to emphasise that you can put together your own routines, alone or with your teacher in class, but always begin with the warm-ups we've suggested.

When you do have a particular need for calm, *Child's Pose* may be the first place to go.

CHILD'S POSE

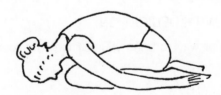

This posture stretches the spine, hips and thighs. It can help to relieve back or neck pain, and encourages the whole body to relax. It is also a deeply comforting *asana,* which can be used at any time you need to rest during practice, or as part of a calming and balancing routine.

1. Kneel with your knees together and your hips on your heels (if this is hard on your knees, use a cushion).

2. Fold forward to rest your chest on your thighs, and try to rest your forehead on the floor. If you have a headache do not drop your head lower than your heart.

3. Let your arms lie by your sides, with your hands by your feet, palms up.

4. If your hips won't reach your heels, or your forehead won't reach the ground, you can make your hands into fists and 'stack' them, resting your forehead on top, or you could use a block or even a thick book! If this is still too much for your knees, lie prone in *Crocodile Pose* instead.

5. Take several deep, relaxing breaths.

If this is comfortable, you might like to try a variation, *Extended Child's Pose*, by placing your hips back on your heels, but stretching your arms far forward, with your hands, palms down, and your forehead on the ground.

You can introduce a practice that uses meditation with this posture, encouraging you to leave behind all the things you have done before – and those you still have to do – to become 'light' and open.

● ● ● ● ● ● ● ● ● ● ● ● ● ● ● ● ● ● ● ●

CHILD'S POSE WITH DEDICATION

This is an excellent way to bring yourself into the room, and to begin a restorative practice.

1. Choose a word or phrase that resonates with you and represents a positive emotion, such as 'I am steady' or 'I am calm.'

2. In *Child's Pose* or *Extended Child's Pose*, and as you are taking your deep breaths, say this word or phrase silently and slowly to yourself. This is your *sankalpa*, or your dedication.

3. Repeat for up to ten breaths as you relax into this posture.

From *Child's Pose* you can move on to the *asana* that asks you to arch your back in graceful movements like a cat.

• •
• CAT POSE
•

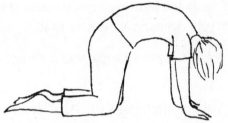

Cat Pose brings flexibility to your spine, while toning and firming your arms and buttocks. But as it encourages you to move with your inhale and exhale breaths, it also soothes and centres.

1. Begin on all fours with your hands shoulder-width apart and underneath your shoulders, and your knees hip-width apart and directly beneath your hips.

2. Inhale, and as you do, lift your tailbone, dip your waist, stretch your throat and look forwards. Relax your belly and let it be soft.

3. As you exhale, round your spine, curl your tailbone under, draw your chin in and push your navel to your spine, holding your tummy muscles in.

4. Repeat for up to ten breaths, with slow, flowing movements, coordinated with your breath.

When you are confident with this posture, you might want to follow with a more dynamic variation that will stretch the sides of your body, prepare you for the twists that will come later, and really get your energy flowing again.

1. In *Cat Pose*, position yourself with a wall to your left.

2.   Extend your right leg in a backward diagonal line from your hip. Feel rooted down into the ground with the outer edge of your right foot. Turn yourself to face right, pressing your left hand firmly into the floor, lifting the right side of the body into a side angle.

3.   Twist to the right, bringing your back against the wall.

4.   Open your chest, and with your right shoulder stacked over your left, stretch your right arm above your head.

5.   Take 5–10 breaths, trying to engage your tummy muscles as you do.

6.   Return to 'neutral', stationary *Cat Pose* for two breaths, then change position so that the wall is to your right, and repeat on your left side for a further 5–10 breaths.

If this feels a bit too much, you could try a short sequence of flowing arm movements with breath called *Hasta Vinyasa*.

HASTA VINYASA

1.   Begin in *Warrior I Pose* (see Chapter 4).

2.   Inhale, and stretch both your arms skywards, pointing up like arrows.

3.   As you exhale, bend your elbows into the *Cactus* position (elbows alongside shoulders, arms bent, palms facing out, like the branches of a cactus).

4.   Inhale, and push up to arrow arms again.

5.   Repeat for five breaths, moving with the breath and feeling the 'responsibility' muscles of your shoulders unglue.

6. Next, with your lower body in the same position, stretch your arms to the sides at shoulder level so that you are in *Warrior II Pose*.

7. Inhale, and make your fingers form cluster buds, like flower-buds, with all the fingers and thumbs touching.

8. As you exhale, flick out your fingers in small, explosive movements, like splashing stars.

9. Repeat for five breaths and try to visualise bright silver stars against a navy blue sky as you do this.

10. Finally, now in *Mountain Pose* (see Chapter 2), with your arms by your sides, palms facing forward and fingertips pointing down, inhale, and sweep your palms up alongside the heart, and turn the palms down.

11. Exhale, and sweep the palms down – as if you are using a paintbrush, and you are painting with the rhythm of your breathing.

12. Repeat five times.

13. Return to *Mountain Pose*, and take several smooth, deep breaths.

14. Now repeat this whole sequence on the other side, beginning with your left leg facing forwards, bending the knee 90 degrees in *Warrior I Pose*.

● ●
● DANCER POSE
●

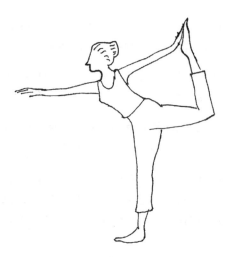

Whichever option you've taken, it would be good to end this part of your practice with a *balance*. This time we'd suggest *Dancer Pose*, which helps you to express yourself with grace and poise. *Dancer Pose* builds lower body strength, and it also requires a steady gaze, a lightness and focus. In time, it will help you to bring your awareness to where you are, so that you are less easily distracted.

1.   Stand in *Mountain Pose* (see Chapter 2) and fix your eyes on a spot in front of you with the soft gaze described in Chapter 3.

2.   Raise your left knee in front of you, then move your foot behind you and try to catch it with your left hand.

3.   Try to keep both hips squared and facing front.

4.   Now raise your right arm in front of you, parallel to the floor.

5.   Gently arch your spine, raise your left leg behind you, open your chest and aim to hold this posture for several breaths, gazing on a still point.

6.   Release, and repeat on the right.

7.   In time, try to hold the pose for ten breaths each side.

Carers told us that one of the benefits of creating time and space for reflection was that they could step back, and respond to situations, rather than react.

JENNY'S STORY ● ● ● ● ● ● ● ● ● ● ● ● ● ● ● ● ●

Jenny is an experienced foster carer, but even she has been challenged by her latest placement, a 15-year-old whose behaviour results in frequent calls from her school.

> 'Most days I'd get a call. She's done this or that. You need to come and get her... With the best will in the world that can get to you, and I'd find myself on the way home saying, what's happened, what have you done now? But I have found a different way. Pause, think about it. Give her some space too... So last time, I took some breaths before I got out of the car. Didn't jump straight in. Let her tell me what had happened. We both seemed better with that.'

Regular practice helped others to come to terms with things outside of their control, and to 'let go' of negative emotions.

MARIE'S STORY ● ● ● ● ● ● ● ● ● ● ● ● ● ● ● ● ●

Marie and her partner came to fostering after retiring, when their children had grown up and left home. They have been looking after two sisters who have been doing very well in their care. Plans have changed though, and it is now likely the girls will return to live with their birth parents. Marie had worried – and even felt some anger – about this decision, even while understanding that it was what the girls said they wanted,

> 'I know the plan is they'll go home. And I know that means that all of the things we'd hoped for, studies, university – especially for the older one - it's not going to happen. But I've got to accept that. Not get too attached. Learn to let go... Being more relaxed about it is helping them too. Helping the older one to be more patient, wait for things to be put in place. Accepting how it is will be best for all of us. Or it could eat you up...'

Twists free and energise the spine and may help us get rid of frustrations that build up when we have to deal with things we may not like, but cannot change. Try a *Floor Doctor* Twist.

● ● ● ● ● ● ● ● ● ● ● ● ● ● ● ● ● ● ● ●

'FLOOR DOCTOR' TWIST

This pose relieves any pressure points in the back, neck and shoulders, and it also (like all the twists below) 'wrings out' the spine like a wet cloth to get rid of physical and emotional tensions that build up there.

1. Lie on your back with your arms straight out at shoulder level, palms up.

2. With your knees pressed together, bring them up towards your chest, and twist slowly to the left. Keep your shoulders on the ground as you do this. Your knees may come to rest on the floor when you do this, but don't force it. It's more important to keep your shoulders rooted than to get your knees down.

3. With your knees on the left, move your head to face the other side – to the right.

4. Repeat on the other side.

5. You can make this a dynamic pose by twisting continuously with your breath – inhale and move your knees to the right, head to the left. Hold.

6. As soon as you are ready to exhale, move back to centre.

7. Inhale, and twist your knees to the left, and your head to the right. Continue for 5–10 breaths.

If this feels good you can try the more intense *Seated Spinal Twist*, with the same benefits.

SEATED SPINAL TWIST

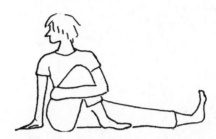

1. Sit with both legs outstretched, lifting your spine.

2. Bend your right knee up and draw your right heel toward your right hip. Maintain a hand's space between your right foot and your left thigh, then hug your left arm around your right knee.

3. Twist to the right, and place your right hand behind you on the floor, looking over your right shoulder. Take 10–20 steady breaths, and then repeat on the left.

Now make a smooth transition through postures to *Mountain Pose* (via *Cat* and *Dog*) to try another standing pose.

TRIANGLE POSE

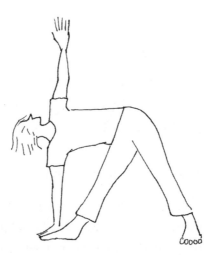

This posture strengthens the thighs, knees and ankles, and by stretching your sides while opening up your entire front body, it encourages a harmonious flow of energy.

1. Stand with your feet 1m (3ft) apart (wider than hip-width).

2. Turn your right foot out at 90 degrees, and turn your left foot in slightly.

3. Stretch out your arms at shoulder level, palms facing down.

4. Take a deep breath in, and as you exhale, stretch to your right, reaching down and placing your hand on your right lower shin without straining. (When you first begin you may need a block to help you if your hand won't reach the floor without leaning forward. Place the block next to your right foot, and rest your hand on top.)

5. Inhale, and stretch your left arm up, turning slightly to look at your raised hand if you can.

6. Hold for several breaths.

7. Repeat on the other side.

And end with another balance. This time you might try *Half Moon Pose.*

● ● ● ● ● ● ● ● ● ● ● ● ● ● ● ● ● ● ●
● HALF MOON POSE
●

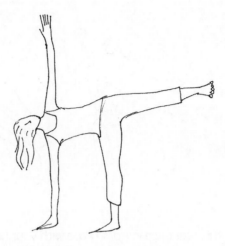

As you stretch, your body will resemble the smooth arc of a crescent moon. It's not easy, but if you practice and find this balance (without fear), it is a feat to celebrate.

1. Begin with feet 1m (3ft) apart (wider than hip-width)

2. Turn your left foot slightly in, and your right foot out at 90 degrees.

3. Bend your right knee, and place your right hand on the floor next to your right foot (or use a block again, and rest your hand on that).

4. Shift your balance to your right foot and hand, and straighten your right leg.

5. Lift your left leg, and stretch up your left arm in the air. Try to hold for several breaths.

6. Lower your leg, and try the balance on the other side.

Liz introduced the Teynham carers to another *Vinyasa*, this time to soothe, ease stress and restore vitality. They sometimes did this sequence to a background of gentle but uplifting music, which they found helped them 'be' with their practice and find the clear-headed quality of *sattwa* (balanced energy). You may like to try this with music too.

● ●
●
A VINYASA FOR SATTWA
●

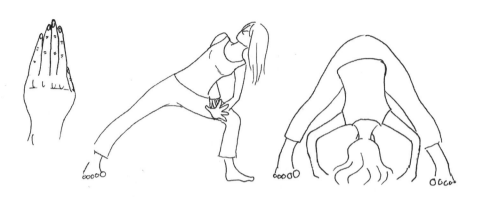

1. Begin this sequence in *Horse Pose* with your hands in *Lotus Mudra*. *Mudras* are gestures, and this one creates the shape of a lotus flower in front of your heart, encouraging communication from the heart. To do this, place your hands in front of your heart, with the heels of your hands, your thumbs and your little fingers touching. Spread your other fingers like outstretched petals. Take four deep breaths, then make the flower into a bud by closing your fingers.

2. With your hands in this 'bud' position, make sure your knees are bending over your third toe, just short of 90 degrees, and begin a dynamic *Horse Pose*.

3. Inhale, and straighten your legs, at the same time stretching skyward with your spine and arms.

4. Exhale, return to *Horse Pose*, pressing the backs of your hands together, fingertips pointing to the earth.

5. Repeat this dynamic *Horse Pose* sequence with the hand gestures for five breaths.

6. Now inhale, lift up your spine, stretch out your arms at shoulder height with your legs wide (left foot turned slightly inward, right foot at 90 degrees and adjusting to make sure your right knee is over the third toe). You are now in *Warrior II Pose*.

7. In *Warrior II Pose* make the 'cluster bud' and 'splashing stars' *Hasta Vinyasa* arm movements with breath we showed you earlier in this chapter. Repeat the movement for five breaths, trying the 'night sky' visualisation as you do this.

8. Then, with your legs in a wide stance, lean your right forearm on your right thigh, into a side bend, with your top arm tucked behind your back.

9. Open your top shoulder and breathe. Look up, or if your neck is stiff, look down.

10. Hold your side bend for ten breaths.

11. Then, adjust back in to a static *Warrior II Pose* for five breaths, followed by a static *Horse Pose* for three breaths.

12. End the sequence on the right with a *Wide-Legged Standing Forward Bend* by adjusting your feet to a wide-legged (1m or 3ft stance) parallel stance. Exhaling, fold forward from the hips, placing your hands on either side of your head. Release your neck, and allow your head to drop. Hold for ten deep breaths for a replenishing 'brain bath'.

13. Repeat the whole sequence on your left side, ending with a final *Wide-Legged Forward Bend.*

Now face the rest of your day with a calm, clear mind.

CHAPTER 7

TIME TO REST

Yoga for Winding Down, Relaxation and Sleeping Well

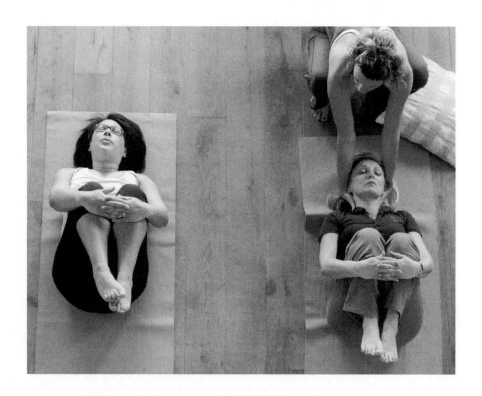

'To the mind that is still, the whole universe surrenders.'[1]

1   Lao Tzu, Chinese philosopher.

Busy carers, whose daily lives may be full of challenges, need to rest their minds and bodies. The carers we've worked with told us that they really looked forward to the final part of their yoga practice, when they could switch off and relax.

BARBARA'S STORY ● ● ● ● ● ● ● ● ● ● ● ● ● ● ●

Barbara has been a foster carer over a number of years, and has looked after young people with special needs who require a good deal of her support:

> 'Just being there helped to clear your mind. Moments when you aren't thinking about what you've already done that morning. Or what you have to do later... And not having to talk or listen. Being peaceful in a room, without having to say anything...
>
> I leave refreshed. Feeling like I've had eight hours of quality sleep. Even when I haven't!'

Whether you are doing your yoga at home or in a class, it's always good to end by winding down, followed by relaxation. Seated poses are generally more contemplative than standing *asanas*, and will help you begin to relax.

When you have completed your routine, you may want to begin this relaxation stage with *Easy Pose*, introduced in Chapter 3.

● ● ● ● ● ● ● ● ● ● ● ● ● ● ● ● ● ●

● EASY POSE WITH PEACE CHANT

This is a traditional meditation pose that encourages restoration after physical exercise as well as soothing the mind and encouraging self-reflection. If you find it more difficult to relax, sitting in this posture and doing simple chanting may help. You can do this on your own, but it works especially well when done with others, and led by a teacher. Try a Peace Chant.

1.   In *Easy Pose*, close your eyes and take a deep breath in.

2.   As you exhale, say the word '*Om*' (pronounced 'aum'), letting the word last as long as your breath.

3.   Repeat three times.

4.   Inhale and as you exhale, sing 'Om shanti (pronounced 'shanty', the *Sanskrit* word meaning 'peace'), repeating 'shanti three times.

5.   Inhale again, and as you exhale, repeat the word 'peace' three times.

Or you may choose to prepare yourself for relaxation by using one of the restorative, supported *asanas*, such as *Supported Fish Pose*.

● ●
●
● SUPPORTED FISH POSE
●

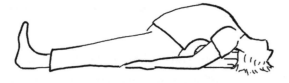

Fish Pose, which we introduced in Chapter 3, is said to have so many health benefits that it is often described as 'the destroyer of diseases'. It gently extends the spine, and makes breathing easier – helping you to settle. When the posture is supported by cushions or bolsters and held for 3–5 minutes, it is especially good for encouraging the mind and body to slow down.

For *Supported Fish Pose* take the position described in Chapter 3, but place a bolster or cushion under the upper back to keep the chest elevated and the head and neck supported. Be careful to keep your body aligned as you would for *Fish Pose*, but as a resting fish you will be able to hold for longer, and really begin to relax.

Another alternative pose that calms you with 'feminine' yin energy is *Shoulderstand*.

· · · · · · · · · · · · · · · · · · · ·
· SHOULDERSTAND
·

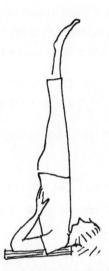

This posture involves the whole body, enhancing blood circulation and soothing the nervous system.

1. It is essential to prepare well, making a broad, firm base by placing a folded rug, towel or four yoga blocks on the floor.

2. Lie with your upper back on the raised base, your shoulders at the edge. Let your head and neck settle slightly lower than your shoulders on the floor. The shoulders are your platform, so don't go any further until you are comfortable there.

3. When you feel stable and ready, gently bring your legs overhead with your hands over the kidney area of your middle back with the fingers pointing upward.

4. Aim to draw your pelvis over your shoulders, extend your legs up and hold as long as you are comfortable, for up to 30 breaths.

5. If this is difficult, you can achieve the same effect in a *Supported Shoulderstand.*

● ●
● SUPPORTED SHOULDERSTAND
●

1.   This time, place a straight-backed chair at the end of your mat and
      a broad, flat padded cushion under your shoulders, with your head
      carefully resting lower than your shoulders.

2.   Holding the chair legs for support with straight arms, slide your
      feet to the front of the chair seat and lift the hips and back.

3.   Raise the knees towards the ceiling, keeping the back of the neck
      relaxed.

Being supported in this way will give you confidence and help you hold the
pose for longer. If you don't have the props, or you still don't feel comfortable,
lying on your back with your legs raised and up a facing wall is a very good
place to end the active phase of your practice. Whichever route you have
taken, you should now be ready for relaxation.

'There is nowhere to go. You are already there.'[2]

The *Corpse Pose* is yoga's quintessential relaxation posture, and usually ends
every *asana* session.

● ●
● CORPSE POSE
●

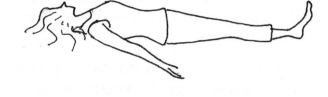

Corpse Pose encourages your mind, body and emotions to settle and
come together. *Supported Corpse Pose* is especially good for producing
a state of deep calm. You should be warm and comfortable, so this is the

---

2   Indian proverb.

time when you may want to put on another layer of clothes or cover your feet with socks.

1. Lie on your back with your legs far enough apart that your lower back feels at ease, feet dropping outward.

2. Let your arms relax away from your sides, palms facing up.

3. Position your head so that you are looking straight up at the ceiling and close your eyes.

4. If you are uncomfortable here, or feeling particularly exhausted, try *Supported Corpse*, which uses props.

SUPPORTED CORPSE POSE

1. Lie on your back as before, this time placing a rolled up yoga mat or a blanket under your knees to allow your lower back to release.

2. Place a yoga block or a folded blanket beneath your head to maintain length through the back of your neck.

3. Whether supported or not, you can now put on an eye mask, wrap yourself in a blanket – anything that will help you to completely switch off.

4. If you are on your own you may like to play gentle music, and simply breathe deeply for 15 minutes or so.

Or you may prefer to use a breathing technique at these moments, such as *Hara (Belly) Breathing*.

HARA (BELLY) BREATHING

Hara (Belly) Breathing centres and boosts self-esteem when you feel physically and emotionally drained.

1. Lying in *Corpse Pose*, breathe gently and focus on your navel. When you first try this, it may be helpful to place your hands on your navel with the fingers touching so that you can feel what happens as you breathe in and out.

2. Inhaling, notice how your navel rises.

3. Exhaling, notice how it falls.

4. Continue until you feel steady and calm, and that your breath is being drawn from within your power centre or *hara*.

You may like to use this time to meditate, use visualisation or even to quietly repeat the word or words you have chosen as your *Sankalpa* or dedication for your own practice. But the Teynham carers particularly valued closing with *Guided Relaxation* led by their teacher when they did their yoga practice together.

● ●

GUIDED RELAXATION

Yoga Nidra is a form of deep relaxation that works best when a teacher guides you. The teacher will give these instructions slowly, clearly and gently, helping you to rest your awareness on each point, and rotate your consciousness around your body. As you do this, breathe softly, and try to imagine each point as a star in a vast and beautiful cosmos.

1. Lying comfortably in *Corpse Pose*, breathe into your eyebrow centre.

2. Breathe into your throat centre.

3. Breathe into your right shoulder joint, right elbow joint, right wrist joint.

4. Now the tip of your right thumb, 2nd finger, 3rd finger, 4th finger, 5th finger.

5. Now your right wrist, right elbow, right shoulder, throat centre.

6. Repeat the sequence on the left side.

7. Now breathe into your heart centre.

8. Now breathe into the right side of your chest.

9. Breathe again into your heart centre.

10. And now into the left side of your chest.

11. Again into your heart centre.

12. Now into your navel.

13. Follow this by breathing into by your pelvic floor centre.

14. Now breathe into your right hip joint, right knee joint, right ankle joint.

15. Now the tip of your right toe, 2nd toe, 3rd toe, 4th toe, 5th toe.

16. Now your right ankle, right knee, right hip, pelvic floor centre.

17. Repeat the sequence on the left side.

18. Now breathe into your root centre, your pelvic floor.

19. Breathe into your navel centre.

20. Now your heart centre.

21. Breath into your throat centre.

22. Now your eyebrow centre.

23. The teacher says, 'Peace. Peace. Peace.'

24. The class repeats silently to self, 'Peace. Peace. Peace.'

25. Follow with three or four minutes of gentle, but uplifting, music. (Classical music, Indian music or Tibetan chants can be very good at these moments as they help the mind let go and relax.)

26. When the music ends, return awareness to the body. After a gentle stretch, roll on to your side to rest, before getting up. *Feel the benefits.*

Ending the day well

JAKE'S STORY ● ● ● ● ● ● ● ● ● ● ● ● ● ● ● ● ●

'We've always done duty fostering which means you can often have a child or young person arriving at all times. And because you might not know them, they don't know the house – the first few nights you'll be alert. Listening out, in case they need something. Or have a nightmare. Or even try to run away. That happens!

The problem is that over time it can affect you. So you find it hard to get to sleep. And even when you do, it's not really deep sleep. You're always kind of "on". And you don't feel properly rested when you get up the next morning, and have to start again...'

Getting a good night's sleep is important for maintaining your vitality, and our carers found that their regular yoga practice helped. But as Jake suggests, carers can find it particularly difficult to switch off at the end of the day. You could try using any of the relaxation poses or techniques we've shown you here, and there are other steps you can take as you prepare for bed.

Let go of the tension

If you have had arguments, disagreements or have had to deal with difficult issues or challenging behaviour (sadly not unusual when you are in this role), try to release any emotional tension when evening comes. Otherwise, your tension can affect your partner or the whole family – creating an atmosphere that makes it hard for everyone to settle down.

End the vicious circle of negative emotions by taking a few moments to release your tensions by lying on your back and placing your feet on an opposite wall – sometimes known as *Legs-Up-the-Wall Pose* – or by trying *Nada Yoga*.

● ●

NADA YOGA

This is the yoga of sound that uses *mantras* to dissolve physical and emotional 'knots' and encourages peaceful sleep. The *Bedtime Mantra* works well.

Bedtime Mantra

In *Easy Pose* (see Chapter 3), quietly repeat to yourself the nerve-soothing *bija*, or seed sound, '*Som*' (pronounced 'sohm') until your body feels heavy with relaxation.

Or to clear a mind racing with too many worries and anxieties, try *Whirlpool Visualisation*.

Whirlpool Visualisation

Sitting in the same pose, imagine a heron sitting by a swirling pool of water. Watch how he disregards the commotion on the surface, only delving into the pool to pluck out life-sustaining fish when the moment is absolutely right – avoiding wasting any energy. Try to do the same by breathing consciously, slowly and 'watching' your thoughts. If you can learn to 'watch', like a heron, you can distance yourself and let them all go.

Leave technology behind

Our phones, tablets, laptops and music players are all supposed to make life easier, and to help us keep in touch with friends and family, but they also keep us connected to our work, can be distracting and even get in the way of a peaceful night's sleep. Carers can feel that they are 'on duty' 24/7 anyway, so although it's tempting to take calls, keep checking emails or messaging, it will really help if you turn everything off at least an hour before you go to bed.

And while you might enjoy having a television in the bedroom (and it may be the only place where you get to see the programmes you really like), this can also be disturbing, especially when you watch a film or a programme that engages or upsets you in any way. So get into the habit of switching off the television when you go to bed. Even try doing this an hour or so earlier with the other gadgets. You may find that, without distractions, you really listen to your partner or family, and it will definitely provide an opportunity to do something that will help you rest.

Give yourself the gift of time

We know it's not easy to make this change, but you will feel the benefits of taking a few moments for yourself to do something you enjoy as you prepare for bed.

You might use this time on your own to do some of the meditation or 'mindful' breathing we have shown you. Or you may want to try an *asana*, such as *Face of Light Pose*.

 FACE OF LIGHT POSE

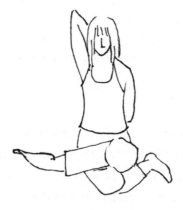

This seated *asana* provides a gentle stretch for your spine, arms and hips, and it also encourages reflection before sleep.

1.   Kneel and drop your hips to the right, crossing your left leg over your right. Your sitting bones should stay on the floor, with your knees forward.

2.   Stretch your right arm over your head, and bend your left arm behind your back, elbow pointing down.

3.   Then bend your upper arm, and reach your hands toward each other, right palm facing in and left palm out.

4.   Hold the pose for five deep breaths.

5.   Repeat on the left side.

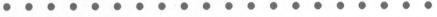

● GRACIOUS POSE
●

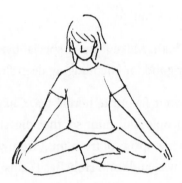

This pose is sometimes called 'the posture of the throne' as its triangular base encourages a noble, yet comfortable, seated position. It is a good way to ground and steady yourself as you get ready for bed.

1.   Sit on the floor with your spine upright, and your legs open wide.

2.   Draw one of your feet in, resting the heel beside your top, inner thigh.

3.   Draw in the other foot and balance it on top of the first.

4.   Rest your hands on your knees, palms downward.

5.   Once you are comfortable, you can practice meditation. Or simply breathe and rest.

Or, after a particularly stressful day, try *Pranic Rest*.

● ●
● PRANIC REST
●

1. Go in to *Child's Pose* (see Chapter 6) and spend the 10 minutes before you go to bed holding the posture and breathing deeply. This will give all your body's systems time to slow down, and bring about a sense of restful equilibrium.

2. Visualising your *prana*, or your breath, moving through your body like soft, golden light as you do this can be especially nurturing.

Or why not use your 'time-out' to:

• Take a relaxing bath. Make it more special by adding perfumed oil. Lavender is very good for encouraging deep sleep.

• Enjoy a cup of your favourite herbal tea. Chamomile is said to aid rest, but some people find mint soothes digestion and makes them feel calm. Add a few sprigs of fresh mint from your own garden. The Indian herbs Ashwaganda and Holy Basil (Tulsi) can also be added to infusions, and they are said to help with sleep.

• Listen to music. Without the television and other distractions you may find you appreciate this more. Experiment with new genres, maybe classical music or jazz.

• Do something creative. Perhaps there is a hobby you've let go, or there's something you would like to take up. It can be very restful to do an activity that is very different from what you do all day. Knitting, needlework, drawing, or even keeping a diary can put you back in touch with yourself, and be very satisfying.

• Simply rest your eyes. Fixing them on a still point and finding your 'soft gaze' can be soothing. And you might use a candle perfumed with rose or lavender as your focus. To keep safe it's always best to avoid having lit candles in your bedroom or around children, and you must remember to put them out. (You can now buy some excellent flameless candles that are just as effective, but without the hazards.)

Remember: It is not strange or selfish to take this personal time. It is absolutely necessary for carers to nurture themselves and to get good rest so that they can keep going. And if your partner and children see you doing these things, you will be setting an example that they may follow. We'll give you more ideas for involving them in Chapter 8.

And so to bed

Calm and relaxed, you should be ready to drift into sleep. But if you find yourself lying in bed still tense and wakeful, there are still things you can do.

LENGTHEN THE OUT-BREATH

1. Breathe slowly and deeply, observing the flow through your body.

2. Gradually lengthen each out-breath until it becomes twice the duration of the inhalation. After a few minutes you will notice how much more relaxed you feel.

Or try a *Sleep-Inducing Mantra, Navel Focus* or *Exhalation Breathing*.

SLEEP-INDUCING MANTRA

Recite very slowly and deliberately to yourself, 'Om hram, om hrim, om hrum, om hraim, om hraum, om hram.'

● ●

NAVEL FOCUS

1. Place your hands on your belly, observing how it rises and falls as you inhale and exhale.

2. This time, as you take ten of these deep breaths, visualise blue-green waves on a gentle ocean, rising and falling with the same regular rhythm.

● ●

EXHALATION BREATHING

1. In these moments of the day, make each exhalation profoundly deep.

2. As you exhale, imagine releasing any remaining physical and emotional tension – let everything go.

3. If you still feel any area of strain or stress in your body and mind, direct your breathing there. Visualise your breath as light, bathing and soothing that area.

Notice how you feel more at peace.

CHAPTER **8**

PASSING ON THE SKILLS

Encouraging Children and Young People to be Healthy

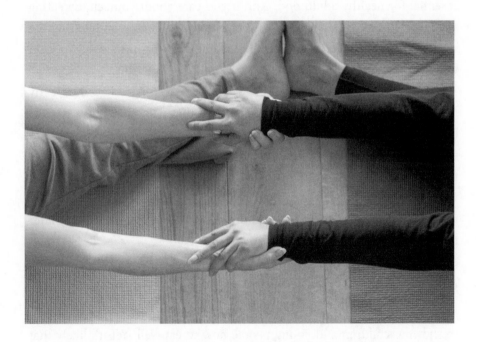

We hope we are inspiring you to look after your physical and emotional health. But there's another good reason for carers to take this seriously. You are bringing up children who are likely to have been through challenging and difficult experiences, and you'll play a key part in their development. Whether you adopt a baby or a small child, are a long-term foster carer, or provide a home for a teenager for a few months, you are a *role model*. This means that the way you live your life, how you cope with stress – even how you feel about yourself and what you do – sets an important example.

If you feel healthy, have confidence and good self-esteem, it's far more likely that the children will grow up with the same attributes. And you will also be teaching them important life skills for a positive future. So in this chapter we present ideas and practices that can be used in everyday life to help you do this. They've been shared by carers, come from our project work or from Liz's teaching with children and young people, so we know they'll make a difference.

Believe in you

Having a strong sense of self – a belief in your own abilities and value – is essential for healthy adulthood. And if you care about yourself, by eating well, doing exercise, managing your emotional wellbeing and getting the rest and sleep you need, then the whole family will be more likely to want to do the same.

But we know many adopted or fostered children have had their early lives shaped by a lack of parental care, and that it is not always easy to break established patterns or to bring about change. Some children and young people may need more specialist help with this, and we'd always recommend talking about concerns and taking advice from your social workers. However, there are things that carers can do to support healthy development and to encourage children and young people to look after themselves.

Encourage healthy eating

Making the simple changes suggested by Alli in Chapter 5 is the first step in showing children and young people how to eat well. Yet it's likely that the children and young people who join your household have been used to something very different. They may have had a limited diet, with only a few familiar foods. They may never have sat around a table as a family to have a meal. They may even have experienced times when there was not enough to eat.

So you might need to go slowly, and you definitely need to be sensitive. With this in mind, try the following:

- Sit down at least once a day together to eat a family meal. This helps everyone to focus on their food (without the distractions of the television or other devices), and it also makes it a social occasion, where they will learn about table manners, and also how mealtimes can be relaxing and enjoyable.

- Involve children and young people in all of the food activities. If they come shopping with you, they can choose new food for the family. They can show you what they know they like, and what they are unsure about. They can help you plan meals. We will say more about cooking and eating together in Chapter 9, but even asking small children to help you shell peas, pick herbs from the garden or stir a cake you're mixing will help develop their interest, and let them see it can be fun.

- Find out about food they shared with their birth family, especially if they are from a different culture or heritage. Showing an interest, and learning to cook this food, will help them feel at home, and also promote a good sense of identity and self-esteem.

- Introduce new food or tastes gradually, by adding a different vegetable to a meal they have eaten before, or making healthier versions of something familiar. You could make a home-made burger with chopped herbs in the mixture and put it in a wholewheat bap – much better than fast-food!

- Make meals that are appealing. Food that is colourful, smells and looks good arouses all of the senses and makes you want to try it.

LINDA'S IDEA ● ● ● ● ● ● ● ● ● ● ● ● ● ● ●

'When our lad came to us we already knew food had been a bit of an issue. In fact, he'd had a few placement breakdowns because he would only eat certain things – and if he was given something else, he'd just refuse. There'd be an argument and he'd go off to his room.

We didn't want to get into those battles. And we definitely didn't want to make separate meals that he'd eat on his own. Food's a big part of our lives and we enjoy eating at home and going out. We wanted him to be able to enjoy that with us.

So we did start making changes in small ways to start. And we did accept that there was a time when it was just chicken nuggets and chips – but I'd get a few peas in somehow! Then we wanted to take a family day trip to France. Go over on the ferry. He was excited about it, but I knew he'd be worried about what we were going to have for lunch.

So I involved him in the planning. Made a list with him about the things he liked. And those he really couldn't face. And most important we came up with a strategy. If we went somewhere and there was nothing on the menu he could eat, then he'd have a drink there, and we'd find a sandwich or a snack elsewhere after.

Well, believe it or not, there was sausage and chips! It was a French sausage and frites – but it was familiar and he was delighted! Tried a bit of salad with it too. And that was a real turning point for us all. He's getting more adventurous and interested now. I still don't push him. But I know he's on his way...'

STELLA'S IDEA ● ● ● ● ● ● ● ● ● ● ● ● ● ●

'We were once looking after a girl who was mixed heritage. She had one grandfather who was Ghanaian, which we are. But she'd never met any of her family from that side and she knew nothing about the culture. I thought that was so sad.

So at weekends we started having family get-togethers. Where I'd play our music. Might even put on some of the clothes with the traditional prints. And of course the food... Chicken and peanut butter soup. Joliffe rice. Some of the fruit or juices...

She liked it. And it opened her eyes to cooking fresh things. Using spices and flavours. But most important it helped her know more about her background. Made her proud of who she is...'

Encourage healthy exercise

This can be a struggle, especially if your child or young person is over-weight or self-conscious. You could try the following:

- Again, seeing you (or your partner or other children) taking care of your body by going to the gym, to class, or practising yoga at home will help.

- You might want to encourage them (if they are old enough) to come to the gym, to go swimming or to a class with you. Some local authorities give special discounts to use their leisure centres or facilities for carers and their children.

- You might have a DVD or a programme they could start using at home until they are more confident.

- You might find that they are more interested in an activity like dance or gymnastics. It could be something you could do together in a class, or they could go to with another of your children.

- Many children and young people who are shy or find it hard to mix relate more easily to animals. So horse-riding might be something to consider. Or even helping out at a stables, on a farm, or walking a dog. If you have an RSPCA or other animal shelter in your area they are always delighted to have volunteers to take the dogs out.

- Or it may start simply by going for country walks as a family. Being in the fresh air, close to nature is something that sadly not all children have experienced.

Remember: Some of these activities can be costly and may be difficult to introduce for that reason. But your agency should be able to help. They may help you find the funds, or they may have their own clubs or groups that your children can take part in.

PETER'S IDEA ● ● ● ● ● ● ● ● ● ● ● ● ● ● ● ●

'We are an outdoor kind of family and like getting out and about – especially in the summer. Getting in the campervan and driving out to the seaside or the country has been part of our son's childhood. But you shouldn't take it for granted that all children have had this.

So when we have a new child we'll always take the van at the weekend with our son and the dogs. And we'll drive out. I might catch a fish. Cook it in the open air. Or even just something you bring with you. Have a picnic and a long walk.

All that fresh air makes you feel good. And you're making a happy childhood memory that they can take with them...'

SANDRA'S IDEA ● ● ● ● ● ● ● ● ● ● ● ● ● ● ●

'I had a 16-year-old who didn't like herself very much. She was heavy. Had lost interest. Spent a lot of time in bed... I admit it wasn't easy to get her motivated but I came up with a challenge. Her mum had mental health issues and there was a charity 10km walk being organised in this borough. I suggested we enter, get sponsored and do it for Mind.

We trained together. And that was not easy for me either! But I was amazed how she stuck with it. And her face when she crossed the finish line and saw what she could achieve was all the reward I needed!'

Encourage a 'healthy' attitude

If you face the world with self-confidence and a positive attitude, you will naturally and effortlessly pass that on to the children you care for. It will also help if you:

- Make an effort to discover what interests them, and what they are good at, especially if they have found school more challenging and are not particularly 'academic'. It may be art, drama, growing vegetables, looking after chickens, knitting a scarf, cutting hair or making a dress. They may surprise you and themselves when you find out what they can achieve!

- Go that extra mile to make pursuing an interest possible. Are they interested in hairdressing? Would your local salon let them go in on Saturdays to help? Or are they enjoying a book they are reading at home or at school? It may be that there is a related film or play. If so, find out where it's showing and take them to see it.

- Explore new things together. There are museums, galleries and parks, and some of them are free. Going out and enjoying these together will encourage their curiosity and engagement with the wider world.

Remember: Your agency and other carers can help. There may be lists of local resources you could have access to, ideas that others can share, and support to find additional funds, if that's needed.

TONY'S IDEA • • • • • • • • • • • • • • •

'I was caring for a group of brothers who had never read a book. In fact, they didn't really understand why anyone would want to read! I came up with this. They liked going on the computer and they liked looking things up. So I said each Saturday, in turns, is your day. We'll go out somewhere different together, to a new part of London where we've never been before.

They loved it! They liked organising the journeys. The buses and trains we'd take. How long it would be. It's true we did spend some Saturdays at the end of the Northern Line...but it got us out, and it got them reading!'

Treat others well

As a carer, what you do, say and how you relate to other people really does matter, and your 'mindfulness' and yoga practice will enhance your awareness – helping you reflect before you react. This is especially important in your relationship with your child or young person. Not only are you setting an example, you are also influencing how they will view themselves for the rest of their lives.

There are things you can do which will build a healthy self-esteem and help them begin to manage their own emotions:

- Make 'special time' when you give them your full attention. We've already encouraged you to switch off your technology and have moments in the day for yourself. We know you are busy, but if you can also tell your child that there are regular periods when you will focus on them, you will all feel the benefits. Switch off or put your phone on silent, turn off the television and do something together that they enjoy.

    For a young child, this might be reading a story or playing a game. For someone older, it might be doing some cooking or going on a shopping trip. A teenager might want to go out for a meal or see a film. Whatever you do, it's just letting them know that you are making quality time to chat or listen – and that it won't be hijacked by anyone or anything else.

- Focus your energy on their strengths rather than constantly picking up on the challenges. And when you give praise for something they've done well, make it specific. If it's some homework they've completed, give a detailed comment. If they've done some tidying up, notice that and be positive. They will feel that you are really interested in what they are doing, and feel valued for their efforts.

- Encourage their problem-solving and independence. We know it's much easier when you're in a hurry to tie up the shoelaces they're struggling with. Or to keep a teenager out of the kitchen because you know the mess that will be made if they make their own breakfast. But if you can let them try a little longer, or live with the disruption, you will be building up their tenacity and allowing them to experience the wonderful sense of achievement we all get when we find we can complete a task ourselves.

- Avoid reacting to a particular behaviour or trigger without thinking about the impact of what you do or say next on the child or young person. We know this isn't always easy, but if you can, take a moment to pause and think, 'Will this bring me closer to, or further away from, the relationship I want with this child?' You will step out of the mundane and it may change your perspective. At the very least it may stop a difficult situation from escalating. And your yoga breathing at these times will definitely help.

- Acknowledge their frustrations and show them you understand how they feel. Sometimes just saying the obvious can have a reassuring effect, 'Oh I can see how disappointed you are...' This simple acknowledgment can help a child feel valued and respected. Over time you will also be helping them to recognise and become aware of their own emotions.

NANA'S IDEA ● ● ● ● ● ● ● ● ● ● ● ● ● ● ●

'I grew up in Nigeria where our grandparents and the village elders told us all of the stories. I'd forgotten about how good it was as a child to sit and listen, and watch them act it all out. It was magical... Then when I started fostering and began looking after children – even older ones – who couldn't read I began my own story telling. With the different voices and the actions and they loved it. And so do I!

Find a quiet time just sitting down together and remembering their favourites or finding a new one. Or even making up a story just for them – that's really special.'

VERNON'S IDEA ● ● ● ● ● ● ● ● ● ● ● ● ● ● ● ●

'One of the boys we looked after couldn't settle at school. And he hated
doing his homework and at times we did despair... But then I found that
we shared an interest in sport. Football, cricket, boxing. Like me he loved
them all. So I decided to try something different. Instead of getting out
his school reading book and telling him to read to me, I'd buy *The Guardian*
or another newspaper. Go into the lounge away from the others and ask
him if he'd like to look at the sport's pages with me. He did, and we'd both
enjoy reading – and then having a discussion (sometimes an argument)
about this or that. I was amazed at how well he could get through that
paper. And it brought us closer together. A bit of "men's time" in a house
full of women!'

SALLY'S IDEA ● ● ● ● ● ● ● ● ● ● ● ● ● ● ●

'The twins I adopted had not had an easy start. And my son especially,
he'd get so frustrated – it would all build up and he'd really struggle to tell
me how he was feeling. Just never been used to doing that. Even scared
to... I thought and thought about what I could do and then I went on this
training where we were asked to look at these pictures of children and
describe what we thought was going on for them. You know, happy if
they were playing. Sad because they seemed on the edge of a group. That
kind of thing.

   I used that but changed it a bit. Instead of photographs I got some
stickers. Smiley faces, sad ones, angry ones. And we had this big calendar
in the kitchen with a kind of whiteboard that I use to organise myself.
You know, a list of appointments, birthdays, etc. for each day. There was
space for a sticker and I encouraged the kids to choose one each morning
and stick it on the whiteboard. I'd do it too. Then before we'd leave in the
morning I could look and say, okay so we're all a bit sad today, I wonder
why? Did it after school as well. And sometimes before they went to bed.
Really helped them to start telling me how they were feeling – without
being put on the spot – and recognising it for themselves...'

This is a similar exercise we've used with carers that could also be introduced to older children and young people.

● ● ● ● ● ● ● ● ● ● ● ● ● ● ● ● ● ● ●

WHAT'S YOUR WEATHER FORECAST?

We're all familiar with a weather barometer as an instrument to predict what the weather will be now and in the future. This practice helps us to learn to recognise our own 'weather' through becoming familiar with the different feeling tones arising in the body. Over time, it can help us to use the body as our own emotional barometer, and we can begin to pick up early signs of particular moods.

1. Identify the part of the body where you most usually feel stress – try to be as specific as you can. Then practice tuning into this part of the body when you feel anxious, worried or any other more 'difficult' emotion.

2. Do the same thing when you are feeling a 'positive' emotion like excitement, calm or happiness.

For younger children and everyone else when you begin, you can use different weather to name the emotions. So feeling 'stormy' may mean 'angry', 'sunny' means 'happy' and so on. You could use stickers or drawings rather than words to express these emotions, as Sally did.

Importantly for you, and your children over time, tuning in this way and noting how a particular emotion affects our body – and then our words, thoughts and actions – helps us make these connections and find a way to manage them.

Finally, practising yoga definitely encouraged some of the Teynham carers to become more aware of their own responses, and to reflect before acting.

JAKE'S STORY • • • • • • • • • • • • • • • • • •

'The 12-year-old with us, now I know he can press all of my buttons! And my wife has said, you can be too hard on him. Some of the things you say make it worse, and you set him off...

But since I've been doing yoga I've learned to take a step back. Take a deep breath in and think about what I'm going to do next before I do it. And my wife has noticed how things are changing between us now, and that there's less of the rows. So we're all feeling better!'

Introducing yoga to children and young people

We can take this further as learning breathing techniques and yoga *asanas* (poses) will help some children and young people to cope with stress, find calm, deal with more challenging emotions and build their own vitality or zest for life.

Guided play for the under-eights

Even at preschool age guided play can begin to focus attention and promote engagement of all the senses. You can try:

- Music: encouraging singing, dancing or playing an instrument. A drum or percussion instrument can be beaten as children move around or strike poses.

- Poetry: speaking or singing simple rhymes, poems or songs – those you know from your own childhood, or new ones you make up! As they get more used to this, the children may learn to chant a simple mantra for positivity, or repeat a phrase to start the day.

- Nature: exploring and getting in touch with nature is of great value to small children. Those who grow up in the city especially need this contact. Squelching in mud, walking in the rain, watching minnows in a river, seeing different insects and animals, hearing the birds...

- Fun: learning and having a purpose are essential, but it's important to balance this with enjoyment and having fun. Show them that even doing household chores doesn't have to be boring if you wash up with lots of bubbles, or dance while you're vacuuming…

Yoga for the over-eights

At eight years old the lungs and immune system are developed, and children are able to concentrate more seriously. So from this age you might introduce simple breathing techniques and chants. From puberty, it's possible to teach all of the main *asanas*, *mantras* or chants and *visualisations*. *Meditation* comes later, usually as a teenager or in the early twenties.

If they see you practising yoga and breathing, it may be that your children naturally want to try. Some of the techniques and practices suggested in this chapter could be introduced at home, but we think it is advisable to involve a yoga teacher, and for your child to attend a class with other children. Careful thought also needs to be given to your child's history and early life. While it can be a real benefit for children and young people who have experienced any kind of abuse to learn about body awareness or positive touch, it does require sensitivity, and may not be the right approach for all.

We think this is something for your agency to consider. It may be that they can set up a group for some children or young people with a teacher who has understanding of their background (as Teynham have done), or it may be that they could help to fund individual tuition for a child or young person who would really benefit.

Here, we present a selection of appropriate postures, sequences and ideas for relaxation. They could be used by a teacher as the basis of a workshop or programme, and adapted for different age groups.

Warm up and wake up

These stretches and poses are preparation for the postures that follow. Once learned, they can be used by children or young people at any time they're out of sorts to feel calmer and happier. Begin in *Corpse Pose*.

● ●
● CORPSE POSE
●

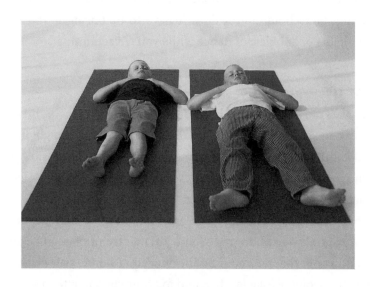

1.   Lie face-up on the floor, with your eyes closed, arms by your sides, palms facing up and toes falling outwards.

2.   Be completely relaxed, so that if a leg or an arm is lifted, it will drop like spaghetti.

3.   Place your hands on your tummy, below your belly button and take a deep breath in. Feel your tummy rise.

4.   Now breathe out. Feel your tummy fall.

5.   Repeat three times, lying as still as you can and letting your mind settle into itself, rather than running into the future or falling back into the past.

Spending a few minutes doing this can fill you with vitality! Next try the *Hedgehog* and *Butterfly* poses.

HEDGEHOG POSE

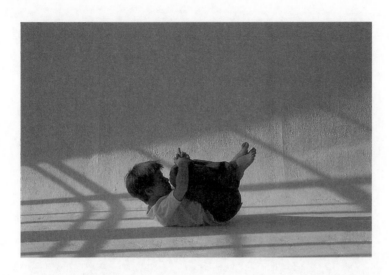

1. Still on your back, curl up, clasping your knees to your chest, and tucking in your chin.

2. Hold for five breaths, then lower your head and legs.

3. Now clasp your left leg into your stomach, stretching your right leg out straight.

4. Squeeze your left thigh into your tummy for five breaths.

5. Change to the right side.

6. Repeat three times on each side.

This stretch will improve balance, massage the tummy and help develop concentration and attention. Then try *Butterfly*.

BUTTERFLY POSE

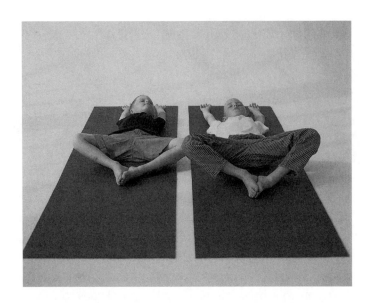

1.   Lie on your back and drop your knees apart with the soles of your feet touching.

2.   Stretch your arms over your head.

3.   Take five breaths.

4.   Flutter your wings like a butterfly (move your legs up and down) to loosen your hips.

You may now be ready to try a linked sequence.

● WAKING UP TO NATURE

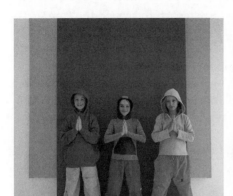 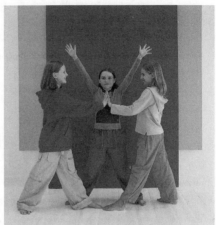

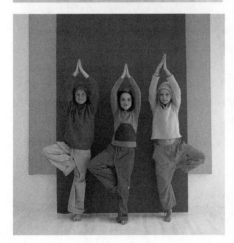 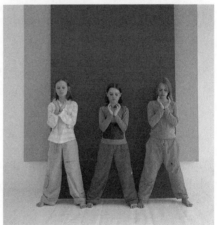

1. Begin in *Mountain Pose* by standing with your legs body-width apart and facing forward. Make sure that your spine is straight and long, like a plant stem, and that your head is lifted towards the sky.

2. Now breathe in and reach your arms overhead like the branches of a tree, stretching your palms and fingers up to the sky. Keep your

feet firmly planted on the ground like the roots of a tree. (If you are working as a group, one person could make the outstretched tree shape while the others form a pattern around the tree.)

3. Now get into *Tree Pose* by standing straight and planting your right foot high on your inner left thigh.

4. Stand rooted into your left foot and stretch your arms straight up like arrows.

5. Look ahead for balance, and take eight deep breaths.

6. Repeat on the other side.

7. Return to *Mountain Pose*, and then cup your hands into the lotus flower *mudra*, so that they look like a large flower-bud.

8. Open the petals (fingers), and look down into the cup of your hands.

9. Take a few deep breaths, imagining the flower-bud opening. Make a wish for your day, and imagine placing it in the centre of the flower.

More sequences to try

You may now be ready to try some of these sequences, depending on age, ability and mood. For strength and bravery, try the following.

PUPPET/RAGDOLL TO WARRIOR 1

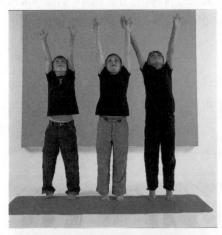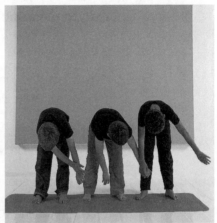

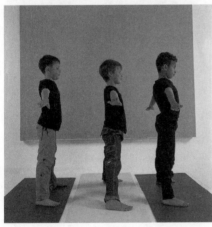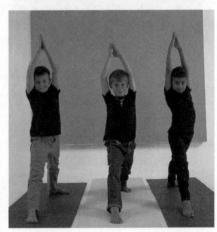

1. Standing with your feet hip-width apart, imagine that you are a puppet. Most of the strings are slack, so relax your shoulders, but feel the string from the top of your head, pulling you up towards the sky.

2. Breathe in and reach up as high as you can, rising up onto your toes. Imagine the puppeteer has picked up the strings attached to your hands, but your toes are still rooted to the floor. Try to feel this deep stretch.

3.   Now flop forward as if you are a puppet or a ragdoll.

4.   Swing from side to side, and as you breathe out make a humming noise, like a willow tree, with breeze moving through its leaves.

5.   Return to *Mountain Pose*.

6.   Take a deep breath and jump your feet apart. Stretch your arms out to the sides, and lift your head skywards to become a five-pointed star.

7.   Raise your arms overhead, with your palms touching.

8.   Turn your left foot in, and rotate so that you turn to the side.

9.   As you breathe out, bend your right leg at the knee, making sure it does not go over your ankle.

10. Hold this pose for five deep breaths. Then repeat on the other side.

You are now rock-steady and focused, like a warrior.

To get rid of tension when you are angry or frustrated, try the following.

● ● ● ● ● ● ● ● ● ● ● ● ● ● ● ● ● ● ●
● LION SEQUENCE
●

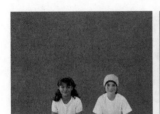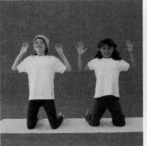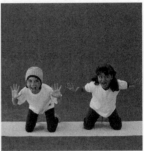

1. Kneel on your mat, resting your hands on your knees, straightening your spine and lifting your chest

2. Lean the trunk of your body forwards and place your hands on the floor beside your knees. Imagine you are a strong lion.

3. Breathe in and grow taller by coming up strongly into a raised kneeling position. Lift your hands as high as your head, and hold them shoulder-width apart. Spread your fingers like claws, like a lion.

4. As you breathe out lean forwards from the hips, open your mouth wide as if to let out a mighty roar and try to touch your chin with your tongue. Stretch your fingertips at the same time, as if you are flexing your claws. Stay here for a few moments and try to empty all your breath.

5. Now put your tongue back in your mouth and relax your face, arms and hands. Lower to a kneeling position, and place your hands back on your knees, back where you started.

6. Take five breaths then repeat the posture four times, trying to grow a little, and become mightier each time you do it.

To refresh the brain and bring calm, try the following.

● ● ● ● ● ● ● ● ● ● ● ● ● ● ● ● ● ● ● ●
● TORTOISE SEQUENCE
●

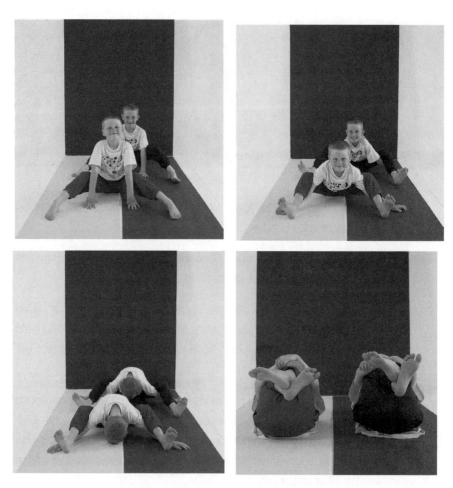

1. Sit on the floor and stretch your legs wide out in front of you.
    Bend your knees slightly. Lift your chest, ready to bend forwards.
    Relax your shoulders and smile, because soon you will be folding
    your limbs around your body to make your own little space.

2.   Bending forwards, thread your arms underneath your knees, so your arms stretch sideways under your legs, a bit like a squashed spider.

3.   Press your palms down and lower your head, trying to press your shoulders to the floor. Keep breathing and stretching out for ten deep breaths. Imagine a protective shell on your back. Close your eyes, and imagine a little cave inside your shell.

4.   Then roll up and slowly gather your arms and legs to your body, clasping your legs with your arms. Roll on your back into a tiny ball, like a sleeping *Hedgehog* (see earlier). Curl up, feeling secure, and take some more deep breaths.[1]

Winding down and relaxing

As in any yoga practice, it is usual to end any session for children and young people with relaxation. These suggestions may be used to close a class, or at other times they may help children or young people relax, and sleep well.

---

1   For more poses, sequences and ideas, please see Lark, L. (2003) *Personal Trainer – Yoga for Kids*. London: Carlton Books Ltd.

INCY WINCY SPIDER

Walking your legs up the wall is a very good way to calm and wind down. Doing it while chanting the *Incy Wincy Spider* rhyme makes it more fun.

Incy Wincy Spider climbed the water spout,

Down came the rain and washed poor Incy out!

Out came the sun which dried up all the rain

And Incy Wincy Spider climbed the spout again.

1. Place your yoga mat against the wall and lie down on your back with your legs resting up against the wall.

2. As you sing the *Incy Wincy Spider* rhyme, begin to walk your legs up the wall.

3. On the second line, run your legs back down, before beginning to climb again on the fourth line.

4. Repeat several times, then rest with your legs up the wall, eyes closed and breathe deeply.

In a group, you might try the following.

SLEEPING STARFISH GAME

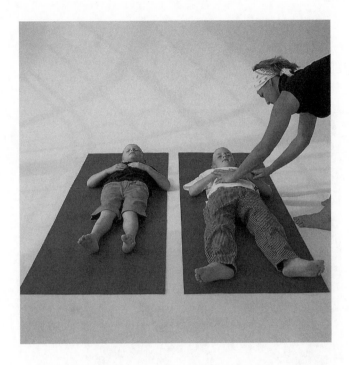

1.   Lie on your back on your mat with your arms and legs stretched out like a huge starfish.

2.   Close your eyes, breathe and try to be as still as possible.

3.   The teacher then walks around and lifts an arm here, or a leg. Touches a nose or ear.

4.   Everyone has to stay as still as they possibly can when this happens – if they move, they are 'out'. The best way to keep the stillness is to focus on the breath, imagining that you are a starfish, not moving or swimming, but staying 'floppy', being carried along by the waves in the sea.

And to close a group practice for children and young people, you might try
Circle Time.

CIRCLE TIME

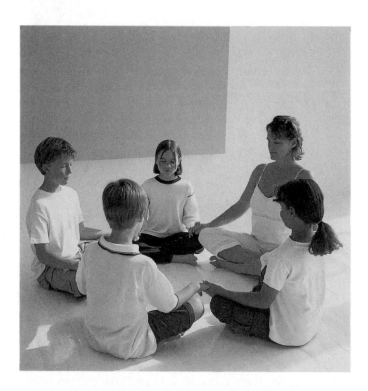

Sitting together in a circle is a perfect way to end a yoga session. It
encourages sharing and a sense of calm.

1.   Sit in a circle, holding hands, with your left hand turned upwards
      and right hand downwards to make a chain, linking hands.

2.   Close your eyes and breathe peacefully, imagining you are
      breathing in through your left hand, and out through your right.

3.   Now open your eyes and reach towards the middle of the circle.
      Clasp your hands together in the middle, keeping your shoulders
      down and relaxed.

4. Breathe in and reach to the sky, fingers interlocked and palms facing up.

5. Now lie back on your mat, put your legs in the air, and make a sculpture by interweaving your legs with others in your circle.

6. Imagine that the wind blows the sculpture over, and flop. Close your eyes, and sleep.

Remember: These postures and games may not be right for older children and teenagers, but they would perhaps benefit most from practising yoga. This always requires careful planning and thought – about the poses and exercises you introduce, group dynamics, as well as the appropriate choice of teacher. We have more advice about how this might work in Chapter 9.

9

IN IT TOGETHER

Supporting Each Other's Health and Vitality

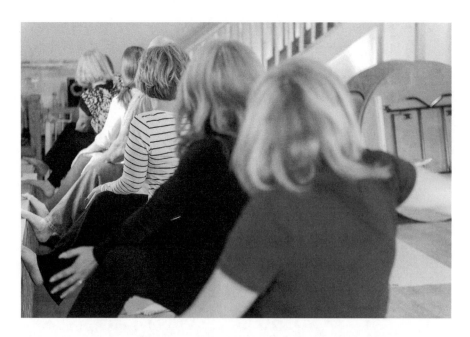

We've been emphasising throughout this book that taking our approach as a family, or even with the support of other carers, can only help maintain your vitality. So here we give you more ideas and tips for feeling healthy together.

Cooking together

There are many ways that carers can get children interested and involved in preparing and cooking good food, such as:

- Start early. Even when children are small they can be encouraged to help by laying the table, doing small tasks in the kitchen, or simply watching what you do.

- Make shopping fun by going to markets, or smaller specialist shops like bakeries or greengrocers, where they can see the variety of fresh produce that's available.

- When they are older a day out to a food market like Borough Market in London where there are all kinds of new things to taste or take home can be very exciting. Even going to a local farmers' market will help make the connection between fresh ingredients and the meals you produce at home.

- Introduce them to growing vegetables or fruit. Small children love the wonder of watching how a seed transforms into something you can pick and eat. If you don't have space, a windowbox is big enough for herbs – even tomatoes. You could find out about getting a family allotment from your local council and grow flowers too. You'll get plenty of fresh air and exercise, and you might even save money.

- Children of all ages love a day out picking strawberries or other soft fruit. Make it even more fun by bringing what you've picked home and using it to make a cordial or a simple pudding like a crumble.

- Show children how to make their own breakfast smoothies with a blender. Even when they are very young you can involve them in choosing and trying different combinations and flavours.

- If they take packed lunches to school, make these interesting by avoiding the same old sandwiches. Add colour and texture, and when they can, encourage them to take an interest and help with this preparation.

- It's really important for older children and young people to have basic cooking skills. Teach them how to make healthy soups, salads, pasta dishes or a stir-fry that keeps costs low. When they're confident, they can try making their 'signature dish' as lunch or dinner for the family. This might become a regular event.

- Buy them their own cookery books and introduce them to different cuisines. There are now some very engaging examples written for children, or better still, written by young people for other teenagers. Show them how to plan a meal from shopping through to presentation. Teaching them to be organised, and to tidy up afterwards, may take a lot of patience and effort – but these are skills that will stay with them.

- In time, cook together. Let them see how satisfying it can be to work as a team in the kitchen.

DAN AND JUSTIN'S IDEA ● ● ● ● ● ● ● ● ● ● ● ●

'We've always had a garden and enjoyed growing our own food. When we moved here, we had the opportunity to have an allotment that we took because it's given us more space. And we've really made the most of it – we've got all sorts now. Potatoes, carrots, runner beans, strawberries, raspberries.

When our 14-year-old came to us he'd spent a lot of time running a bit wild. His parents doing their own thing really... He didn't have a clue about how to look after himself and of course knew nothing about vegetables! But he's an outdoor kind of lad, and he always liked to come and help us digging, planting, a bit of weeding...

Dan's always done most of the cooking and he's very good at it. In fact, his mum's a chef. So he's always used what we've grown. And our lad started taking an interest in that too. Showed him how to make a runner bean chutney (which is good with cheese or a salad) and raspberry cordial – which you can freeze in the summer for granita.

It's been really rewarding to see how he's come on with this. He's thinking of his own ideas too – and he's showing a real flair. So we're going to try and help him get his work experience next year in a restaurant we know. 'Cos he definitely enjoys it all and he says he's thinking about cooking as a career...'

JACKIE'S IDEA ● ● ● ● ● ● ● ● ● ● ● ● ● ● ● ●

'I had a teenage girl who really worried me. I knew she'd be leaving care soon, but she had spent a lot of her childhood in a children's home where they weren't allowed anywhere near the kitchen. So how were they supposed to know about cooking for themselves?

When I was younger I was in the Women's Royal Air Force – in catering, actually. In charge of a canteen. And I brought that experience to my fostering. It's been really useful with teenagers because sometimes it's a different kind of parenting they need. More focused. Teaching them things. Breaking it down into tasks, small achievements, and then moving on to the next. Because you know that before long they are going to be out there on their own, and they really need to be able to manage...

So with this girl I set her a task. To plan and cook her own lunch for a week when she was off college. Gave her a budget too. First time we tried she blew it all in the first couple of days. Bought a lot of convenience stuff, crisps, sweets. So we went back to the drawing board. Helped her plan, think about where she'd get the best bargains. How she could make something, have some things left over and then she could use that in what she made the next day. All those things you learn when you're in catering.

Once we'd cracked that we moved on to planning all of our meals. Then she organised her own birthday party. Everything she chose and wanted – again, managing what it all cost. And each thing she got right meant her confidence grew. And I found out what she could do, and what we needed to do more work on.'

THE SANKOFA STORY ● ● ● ● ● ● ● ● ● ● ● ● ● ●

Sankofa care is an independent fostering agency in South London. They were concerned about too many young people leaving care without the ability to cook, and wanted to do something about it. So they asked Andrea to lead a project with some of the teenagers they had in placement.

Andrea did focus work with the teenagers, asking them about what they liked to eat, what skills they thought young people need, and their own ideas for encouraging teenagers in care to eat healthily.

She then brought in a chef who ran a day workshop showing them how to prepare and cook their favourite meals, and who taught them the basic skills. Sankofa used this material, including the recipes, information and tips, to make a publication they called *Cook Up!* They presented a copy of *Cook Up!* to all of their foster carers during Fostering Fortnight that year, providing a tool they could use *with* their young people.

Eating together

It's so important for children and young people to understand that eating good food meets more than just physical needs, especially if they haven't had positive experiences of family life. Getting together over a meal can be a *social* event too – it can be fun. It doesn't need a lot of fuss, and it's a great way to say thank you, to celebrate a birthday or an achievement. And it can show a friend who's feeling down that someone cares.

- Introduce children who join your household to family traditions – maybe one night a week when you get together to enjoy a big pot of curry, or taking it in turns to make the evening meal for each other, or a particular dish you eat on special occasions. If you don't have these 'rituals', create some together!

- Are there dishes or food traditions that your child or young person can introduce to you? If they have a different heritage or background, ask them to tell you what they know, and show the rest of the family. There may be celebrations like Diwali, Chinese New Year or Independence Days that have associated foods and meals. They may become an established part of your family's traditions too!

- Encourage them to be social – inviting friends for tea. Later on they may want to ask a small group to cook and eat something simple together at home. Pancake parties (with a choice of fillings) always work well – with some supervision and support of course!

- Celebrating birthdays is something we all take for granted, but sadly this may not be part of every child's past. So make sure you mark these events. Making and sharing a birthday cake can be a lot of fun, and can help a child or young person feel special.

SHABNAM'S IDEA ● ● ● ● ● ● ● ● ● ● ● ● ● ● ● ● ●

'I'll never forget our son's first birthday – his eighth – that he celebrated here with us. He had never had a proper party – even a cake. When I realised, I went out of my way to do something he wouldn't forget. We looked in books, went on the internet. And he chose a cake he wanted. But I didn't want to just go out and buy something. As it turned out it wouldn't have been possible anyway as he wanted a rocket. In purple. His favourite colour at the time!

So we made it together. My daughter who was 12, and has always loved baking, joined in too. It took all morning, there was mix everywhere by the time we'd done. But that evening, lit up with candles it was magical...

We still do it. He's 16 now but each year we'll make his birthday cake. Last year it was a Red Velvet – not as ambitious as the rocket maybe – but he was just as proud!'

THERESA AND JOHN'S IDEA ● ● ● ● ● ● ● ● ● ● ● ●

'We look after a lot of teenagers and getting them used to cooking is always a priority for me. But it can be an uphill struggle, so you've got to make it something they want to do. So for the past few years we've been doing "cook offs"! What are they? They come from something that used to be on the telly. Two teams. One headed by me, one by my husband John. We have to do a dinner and pudding on a Saturday night with everything fresh. From scratch. And my long-suffering nextdoor neighbours get to eat with us. Then they decide who's the winner... It is such a laugh, it really is. But at the same time they are learning.'

Cooking and eating with other carers

Getting together to share a meal can also provide a valuable opportunity for carers to meet – and to support each other. It might be something as simple as having coffee (or maybe a herbal tea!) in each other's homes. But there are some agencies that take this more seriously, and organise events around meals to facilitate carer meetings, or even as a way to show that they appreciate what you do:

- Having a meal or going out to lunch together is a sociable way to connect with other carers and to share experiences – without necessarily having to focus on problems or difficult issues. This may be more uplifting and energising for everyone involved.

- Or it may be that you prefer something informal, arranging to bring a simple (healthy) dish that you then eat together. Or in the summer months, a barbeque with everyone contributing and involved in the cooking is especially fun.

- It is important for agencies, or those who work with carers, to think about how they might help. Providing a venue or funding an event like this makes an important statement.

JAKE AND DEBBIE'S STORY   •   •   •   •   •   •   •   •   •   •   •

Jake and Debbie have been foster carers for a number of years. Their agency organises group supervision every fortnight at their local centre. If they choose, carers can bring a dish, and use some of this time to meet and talk with each other. The attractive building has a light and spacious kitchen so they can also cook lunch there, eating around a large table or outside if the weather is good. The centre manager funds these lunches and sees this as an important part of the support they provide. Jake and Debbie really value this provision.

'We are always busy, that's true. But we do make time for our Thursday lunches. We'll have a curry, salads. Good homemade food. And it's a chance to talk things over if that's what you want. Or you might not want to discuss the kids or any issues at all. You might just want to get away from some of it for a bit – time off, if you like. Being able to be yourself.'

Practising together

We also believe that coming together to practise the breathing and yoga *asanas* we have introduced in this book can be an additional source of support for some carers. Again, agencies could supplement your home practice by providing a venue and a teacher to make this possible.

Jake and Debbie are Teynham carers, and their fostering agency piloted our project, funding Liz's yoga sessions over ten weeks, with a positive impact on the carers' health and wellbeing. The participating carers also told us that practising in this way helped them feel part of a 'community'.

JAKE'S STORY ● ● ● ● ● ● ● ● ● ● ● ● ● ● ● ●

'Adding the yoga before our Thursday lunches. Well, I was a bit sceptical to start with. But I wanted to do more exercise so I gave it a try. And I'm so glad I did. There was just something about being in a room with other people. Doing something together. Not having to say anything. Not having to talk even. But knowing you are there with people who understand.'

Yoga may not be for everyone, but there are other things that you can do together that will help maintain your vitality and keep you engaged with the wider world:

- Going for regular swimming sessions or other exercise classes. Some local authorities provide free or subsidised membership of leisure centres for their foster carers.

- Learning to dance. There is a range of possibilities in most areas now. Salsa – not too difficult to learn and very upbeat – is a good choice.

- Getting an allotment or gardening as a group. Ask your agency to make enquiries with the local authority as you may have some priority for one of their spaces.

- Sewing or other crafts. Is there something – a quilt? Cushions? Something your children or young people could use that a group of carers could make together?

- A pottery or art class. Most adult education centres run a variety – or maybe your agency would pay for a teacher at a time that suits you.

- A book club. But try to avoid the temptation to only choose novels or stories about social care issues.

- Go out as a group to visit a gallery or an exhibition. It may give you ideas about things you can do with the family, but it may also revive interests you've let go.

- See a film or go to the theatre – maybe a musical or a show. A matinee when the children are at school is a possibility, and tickets will usually be cheaper then too.

- Some carers have become campaigners, identifying a shared need in their support groups and then thinking about what they can do to bring about change. This takes them away from individual worries and problems, and helps focus their energy on an achievable goal.

Yoga for groups of teenagers and young people

In Chapter 8 we suggested introducing yoga to children to promote their good health and wellbeing. Organising a group for teenagers where they'll learn some of the breathing techniques and simple poses can be particularly beneficial, especially if their early lives mean that they struggle to manage their emotions, have trust issues and may not feel very good about themselves.

This clearly does require great sensitivity and careful planning, and you'll need an excellent teacher who understands their particular circumstances and issues. But we did try this in Teynham with some positive results.

THE TEYNHAM STORY ● ● ● ● ● ● ● ● ● ● ● ● ● ●

After piloting yoga for foster carers, the Teynham centre considered setting up a group for some of the young people they were looking after. Following discussions with Liz they decided that this would involve a very small number of 14- to 17-year-old teenage girls, whose carers were already doing yoga themselves. They didn't know each other at the outset, but for a number of reasons they all had low confidence and poor self-esteem.

The girls began with some input from Alli, our nutritionist, and they did some cooking together with her – sharing the meals they had prepared. Once they were more comfortable with each other, Liz thought very carefully about the exercises and techniques she would introduce, as well as her style of teaching. She always kept the yoga sessions relatively short (40 minutes), light and fun. And she always noted and stopped anything that seemed to make anyone in the group uncomfortable.

The girls responded well, and said they liked the breathing and the relaxation part of the sessions. They also enjoyed being with each other, and doing some simple partner work as part of their practice.

We would encourage more agencies to think about what might work for a group of their young people. We present a few ideas from our Teynham pilot here, but a skilled teacher could adapt any of the breathing, visualisation, poses and sequences from previous chapters. You'll find more ideas for group work in Liz's book.[1]

Yantra breathing

A *yantra* is a pattern, often geometrical, that is used to help the mind concentrate and focus during breathing and meditative sessions. Introducing a tangible symbol – either a square or circle – helps young people to connect to their breath. Try this *Breathing with a Square* to calm and centre.

---

1   See Lark, L. (2003) *Personal Trainer – Yoga for Kids*. London: Carlton Books Ltd.

BREATHING WITH A SQUARE

1. Visualise a square in your mind's eye. (With children or young people, it works best if the teacher draws and cuts out a square shape (30cm/12in) from coloured paper, then tapes the square to a wall at eye level, and asks the group to sit in a comfortable cross-legged pose, with their spine straight in front of it.)

2. Gaze at the bottom-left corner of the square. Breathe in and trace the line with your eyes to the top left-hand corner.

3. Breathe out, following the line with your eyes, and breathe from the top-left corner to the top-right corner.

4. Breathe in, following the line with your eyes, and breathe from the top-right corner to the bottom-right corner.

5. Breathe out, following the line from the bottom-right corner to the bottom-left corner.

6. Repeat this exercise five times.

Or you may want to try a more active exercise, which we used in Teynham. It is good for coordination, but as it involves working with a partner it can also build trust.

MIXING BOWL

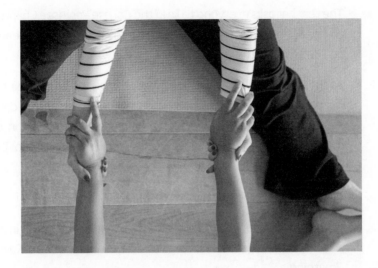

1.   The teacher divides the group into pairs and asks each pair to sit facing their partner with their legs wide and stretched out in front. The four legs should make a square, with the soles of the flexed feet pressing against each other, palms of their hands resting on the floor.

2.   The teacher asks each pair to clasp hands with their partner, keeping their arms straight. Then they begin to stir a circle round and round – as if they were mixing a huge pot of dreams, but making sure they are coordinated and circling in the same direction!

3.   They keep circling from side to side and forwards and backwards, trying to keep the movement flowing and fluid, and think about what's in their pot. What are they mixing? They should tell the teacher when she comes around to check on their cooking.

You could also try a visualisation, which can be good as part of relaxation for young people in a class, but then can also be used on their own to get to sleep at night.

RAINBOW BATHING

1. The teacher asks everyone to lie in the *Corpse Pose* (see Chapter 7), to close their eyes and imagine their body is floating like seaweed on the sea, and to breathe deeply.

2. As they lie floating in warm, aquamarine water, they imagine there is a broad rainbow above their heads, and see the rainbow colours as they imagine them to be – one by one – and bathe in each colour. Red... Orange... Yellow... Green... Turquoise... Deep blue... Pink... Purple... Gold...

3. They should feel the quality of each colour and breathe it in.

4. Then they pick their favourite colour for today and bathe in it for a few moments (the teacher gives one minute of silent *Rainbow Breathing*).

5. Then, very slowly, they begin to wiggle their fingers and toes. They begin to stretch out their faces, and give a big body 'yawn', stretching out in all directions.

6. Now slowly, and in their own time, they sit up, noticing how refreshed they feel having visited their own special place.

Closing practices

To end sessions with older children and young people it may work to introduce 'closing time'. The teacher might read a poem, play a piece of music or even encourage singing together. But you don't want to make anyone feel out of place or uncomfortable, so you have to think carefully about your own young people and what will work for them.

Introducing yoga or any of these practices will require careful thought and extra effort to understand the needs of the young people involved. But if you make this effort, the long-term benefits for their confidence, health and wellbeing as they move into adulthood will make it worthwhile.

CHAPTER 10

KEEP ON KEEPING ON

Being a Healthy Carer

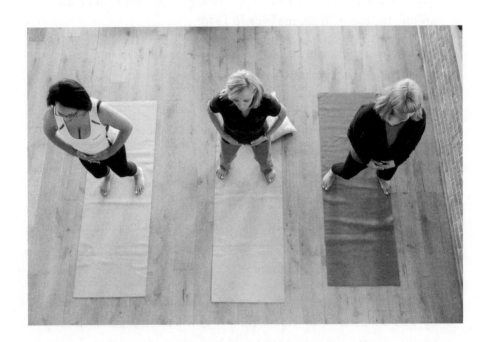

'The root of compassion is compassion for oneself.'[1]

Finding vitality is one thing, but keeping that zest for life is the real challenge, especially when you experience the daily demands of being a carer. The

---

1   Pema Chodron, Buddhist teacher, author, nun and mother.

support of others does help, but in the end you have to find your own way to maintain a healthy self and keep going.

Over the years, Andrea has heard lots of stories from carers about what they do when things get difficult.

When the going gets tough

'We pack our bags, load up the campervan and take off for the coast. The whole family. Just a day away, that change of scene – puts it all in perspective.'

'Get my headphones on, Bee Gees *Saturday Night Fever*, and dance around the room. Takes me back to 1976…'

'Have a long soak…the full works. Bath oil, candles. Even take in a magazine. A whole hour to myself.'

'We will take some respite and get away together. Just my wife and me. Somewhere sunny and warm with a good beach. And no children… That's our time.'

'Do some DIY. No seriously! I'm dyslexic but I've always been really good at making things. And I teach myself. My husband used to laugh, but last year I tiled the whole bathroom. Did a fantastic job – so he's not laughing anymore. And it's so different from what I do every day, it just clears my mind.'

'Call my mum. She was a foster carer too, and she brought six of us up. She just listens and lets me rant. And when I'm done she'll say, okay. Get some rest now. Then you'll be ready for tomorrow…'

'Take the dog out. Watch her run through the fields, enjoying herself. Her energy gets mine back!'

'Sky sports!'

'Spend a day with my sister. Doing the glamorous things that she does. And have a laugh of course. I come back with a fresh take on things!'

'Used to go to the gym, but now it's yoga. My weekly class keeps me going, but in between, just five minutes every morning doing my breathing makes all the difference...'

DOING IT JAKE'S WAY ● ● ● ● ● ● ● ● ● ● ● ● ● ●

Jake and his wife Debbie are Teynham carers, and taking part in our yoga pilot had quite an impact on them:

> 'When I was a mechanic and I worked with cars, I'd teach the apprentices. Sometimes they'd say, "you're doing it wrong – he told me to do it like that." So I'd say, "Listen. You'll learn from me, and you'll learn from others and you'll find the way that's best for you..."
>
> Fostering's like that too. Over the years you try a bit of this, take a bit of that. Find what works for that child and you at that time. All I know is that you won't find the answer in a manual or a textbook...
>
> And now with the yoga it's something else I have. Another tool if you like. It can calm me, make me take a bit of a step back. Let the frustrations go about things I can't change. But someone else might use it differently. That's okay 'cos in fostering you have to find your own way – and this will help you find it.'

Not all of the carers we've worked with have embraced the ideas presented in this book to the same degree as Jake, but they all now have enough understanding to add these techniques to their personal coping strategies, *and* to use them if and when it feels right. Some of the carers have gone on to make significant changes to their lifestyle, while others have found improving their diet or using a particular breathing technique is what works for them.

Our intention has been to encourage you and those who support you to open your minds and to consider taking a different approach. And in this final chapter we suggest how yoga practices will keep you doing what you do well.

You may decide to add our ideas to the things you already use, or we may have inspired you to take a fresh look.

What an agency can do

- Start taking the wellbeing of carers seriously. We don't mean becoming fixated on things like a carer's weight, but we do think you should take an active interest in their physical *and* emotional health, and review it over time.

- Take a look at the support you currently offer to keep carers healthy. Yes, you may facilitate support groups, but do they work for everyone? Some carers tell us they feel 'talked out', and that as these groups inevitably focus on the children's problems or difficulties, they can leave drained – more tired than when they arrived. Think about adding something new.

- What are you doing to support carers' role in teaching children and young people the vital life skills they need for adulthood? It's not just a case of knowing how to cook or budget; they need to be emotionally 'ready' too, and the adults who bring them up are their most important influence. Think about what you offer to help carers manage their own emotions and to pass on these skills.

- All carers need to take a break and make time for their family, partner and self. This is essential to remain positive, and to have the energy to provide the good quality care that is so badly needed. Do you encourage them to do that? And do you have a respite system in place that makes this possible? We know that social workers are often concerned when carers want to take a break or holiday without the children they are looking after, but this can be managed, and there are some excellent practice examples to draw on. If children know their respite carers well and understand how this works, it can be a positive break for them too – like going to stay with a grandparent or an aunty.

- Encourage and support carers to make time in their daily routines for doing something – whether breathing, meditation or simply sitting in the garden – which nourishes them.

- Consider how you contribute to creating a carer 'community'. Do you provide opportunities for them to come together socially, and to do things that don't relate directly to their role? Could you help facilitate a lunch club, outings, a gardening group, something that isn't necessarily focused on the children but that brings carers together?

- Do carers see that you value them and what they do? You may have award ceremonies, or appreciation days, but is this enough? How are they treated by the agency? Are they really listened to, and do staff show an interest in them as individuals? If they know that you are concerned about their health and wellbeing, they're more likely to feel good.

- *Think about providing our programme for new and established carers.* Coming together and being led by good teachers like Liz or Alli is the best way to introduce the yoga practices we've presented here. If you do make this investment, carers will be equipped with new coping strategies, they will be more likely to stay energised and motivated, and you will be making a very important statement about your commitment to looking after them.

THE TEYNHAM APPROACH ● ● ● ● ● ● ● ● ● ● ●

Andrew manages the regional centre in Teynham that piloted our programme with foster carers. He has been involved in the fostering world for many years, and has always believed that agencies have a responsibility for carers' wellbeing.

'Fostering, of course it can be difficult. And it can be lonely... Here there's a lot of looking after very troubled young people when it's only the carers' determination that sees it through.

But it doesn't have to be like that. I believe that we should help. And that's the way we do it here at Teynham. I've brought our carers together for the Thursday lunches for that reason. It's part of making a community. Saying that you're not on your own in this. We also have a children's group one evening a week. Which we set up because lots of the children couldn't fit in at youth clubs, things like that. We have workers who organise the activities – and that frees up the carers to have a break, spend some time with each other. Because I do encourage them to take breaks. It makes sense, doesn't it? What good are they to me or the children if they are tired, worn out, with nothing left to give?

When I heard about the yoga I was very willing to try that too. For the same reason. Anything that might help carers do what they do I will try. Of course, costs matter. But for me, this is all part of retention. Finding and recruiting carers – that's the easy part. Keeping the best ones is the challenge. And my carers are definitely worth investing in!'

What you can do

- You may not be ready to follow all of Alli's principles (see Chapter 5), but you can become more aware of how and what you eat. Notice if some food makes you feel bloated or sluggish, and whether there is any impact on your energy levels or mood. Listen to your body and make the changes that it's asking of you. And if you don't already, have proper times – at least once a day – when you sit down as a family together, without any distractions, and enjoy your meal.

- Introduce regular exercise into your routine. This might be going to the gym, but it could be anything that suits you – dancing, swimming. Or best of all, go for a walk, with the added benefits of being outside in the fresh air. Take more interest in your physical health, and notice the difference that even a small effort makes to how you move and how you feel.

- Find something that you enjoy doing which will give you a break from 'caring'. Rediscover a hobby, or find a new one. Try to make it something that takes you away from the problems and issues that may be part of your everyday life, and that brings out your creative side.

- Make time for your family and your partner. If you can, take regular breaks to focus on each other. And most importantly, take time for yourself. We know that this may be easier said than done, but introducing even a few moments each day to simply be will bring long-term health benefits. This isn't selfish – it's absolutely necessary!

- Use mindfulness to become more aware of your emotions and how you are feeling. Take note of your mood and your thoughts, especially the more difficult ones. Tune in to your body, and notice the connection between these feelings and the physical sensations they produce. In time, you will be able to notice signs or symptoms of becoming angry or overwhelmed, and you will be able to use some of the techniques we've shown you to pause, slow down, take a rest…

- Relaxation and plenty of sleep are very important. You need to find your way to 'switch off', and if your sleeping pattern becomes disturbed, you should always take this seriously and seek advice.

- If you are struggling and it seems like you're on your own, talk to the team. It may be that your agency can introduce you to other carers, or that they organise groups or activities you can join. If you don't think they are listening, or they don't offer support, think carefully about your options. As Andrew says, if *you* aren't feeling good and *they* don't take this seriously, how can you care for others?

- And, of course, the yoga we've presented in this book has been chosen to take all of these needs into account, and to nourish your vitality. If you practise regularly on your own – or even better, as part of a routine that includes a class – you'll find the physical, mental and emotional balance to be a healthy carer. You'll also be such a good role model for the children and young people you're bringing up.

To end, we would like to give you suggestions for short, simple practices that could become part of your daily routine. These won't take too long, and you can do any of them at home – taking a little time out every day to *take care of yourself.*

Take just ten minutes for a *Sun Greeting.*

● ●
●
SUN GREETING
●

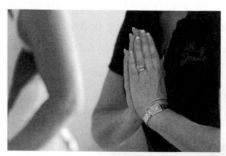
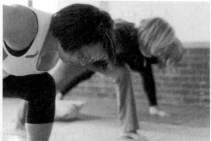
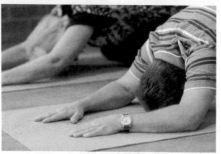

Surya Namaskar, or sun salutations, are a short sequence of movements from classical yoga that wake up the whole body and generate energy. Repeating several of these sequences every day will strengthen the heart, detoxify and revitalise all of the systems. And on a subtle level, they also balance your left and right nerve channels, encouraging steady emotions and a calm mind – helping you to keep going.

1.   Begin in *Mountain Pose*, feeling the four corners of your feet rooting into the earth. Rock back and forth to find the balance of even weight between the front of your feet and your heels. Place your hands to your heart and take a full deep breath.

2.   Breathe in and sweep your arms wide, circling them up to the sky and meeting the palms above your head. Stretch up.

3.   Breathe out and fold over the front of the hips into a forward bend, bending the knees softly to avoid back strain. Drop your head like a heavy bell. Then, if you can, place your hands on the floor.

4.   Breathe in and lunge the left foot back, dropping the left knee onto the floor, creating a lunge and stretching the hips. Breathe deeply out.

5.   Breathe in and step the front (right) foot back to join the left, so you are in a high plank position, with the legs together, the arms vertical like two strong pillars. Hold this position and take another breath in, opening the chest and drawing your shoulder blades down the back.

6.   Breathe out, and gently lower your knees, chest and chin to the floor, and rest in *Child's Pose*.

7.   Come back to *Mountain Pose* and repeat all of the steps on the other side (beginning by lunging the right foot back).

8.   Do this sequence three times on each side. You can take a rest in *Child's Pose* between each sequence if you need to. You may want to build up to doing five or even ten sequences, but always remember to do the same number on each side to keep the body balanced.

Traditionally *mantras* were recited during sun salutations, matching movement with sound. You could try singing mantras with each step, which distribute *prana*, or energy, through the mind as well as the body.[2]

---

2   See Lark, L. (2015) *Creative Yoga Practice*. Available to purchase at www.lizlark.com/creative-yoga-practice-book.

Take five minutes for *Makkho-Ho Stretches.*

• •
•
• MAKKHO-HO STRETCHES
•
This short sequence of movements come from classical Chinese medicine, and is said to balance the six pathways of energy (or 'chi') in the body. There are six movements, which each relate to a different body part, and harmonise each of these pathways to let the energy flow. At the same time they also balance *yin* and *yang*, concepts from the traditional Chinese belief system that relate to the 'masculine' and 'feminine' sides of our nature. Again, regularly doing these six stretches will provide the physical and emotional resources you need to 'top up' and nourish your vitality.

1.   Start with a *Standing Forward Bend*. With your legs body-width apart and both feet pointing forward, fold from the hips, and let your head hang like a bell. If you can, straighten your legs, but if this is difficult, keep your knees soft. Let your arms fall to your sides, or raise them up to point to the sky if your shoulders allow. Take a deep breath.

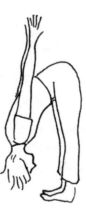

2.   Next, move towards a *Reclining Hero Pose*. Kneel on your mat, and place your palms on the small of your back. Lean into a backward bend. If you are in this position you can reach your arms over your

head so that they lie on the floor behind you. If this is too difficult, you can lie on your back with your knees raised and feet on the floor, hip-width apart. In this position raise your arms over your head and rest them on the floor. Wherever you are, take a breath.

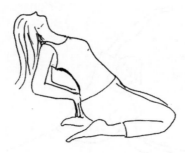

3.   Now sit up in *Butterfly Pose* by sitting with your spine straight, your feet in front, soles touching, so that your legs make a triangle shape. Place your palms together at your heart and take a breath.

4.   From there, stretch your legs straight out in front of you with your feet flexed. Bend from the waist into a *Seated Forward Bend*, holding your feet if you can, or placing your hands as far down your legs as is comfortable. If this is too difficult to do with your legs stretched out, you can bend your knees and avoid rounding your back. Take a breath.

5.   Now sit back up into a cross-legged position and bend forward with your head down. Breathe.

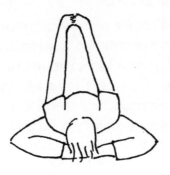

6.   Finally sit with your legs wide in front of you. Reach up with your
        left arm, then move your upper body to the right, with your arm
        close to your head and ear into a side bend. Take a breath, and
        then repeat for one breath on the other side.

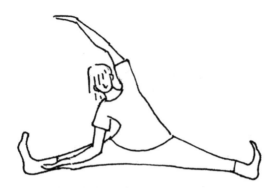

You will become more flexible as you do this more often, but never push your
body or force it into uncomfortable positions. Make your own adaptations
if you need to.

If you feel you have no time for this, are worried about doing anything
too physical, or even if you're sceptical about our approach, we hope we can
persuade you to use this *one* simple technique.

Take just a few moments to do this *Mini Hasta Vinyasa*.

● ●

● MINI HASTA VINYASA (SITTING AND
● MOVING WITH THE BREATH)

Breath can be an anchor for people with stressful lives, and if you only
bring mindfulness to your breathing, it will steady and ground you. But if
you are someone who finds it hard to sit still to do the breathing exercises
we've shown you, or if you can't focus with so many thoughts racing
through your head, bringing some movement into your sitting might help.

If you feel yoga is really not for you, we still ask you to take a little time
daily for yourself to do this simple breathing practice. We know that even
this small change will make you feel better.

1. Sit in a comfortable seated position – *Easy Pose* is good (see Chapter 3) – with your hands in your lap, palms up. Or if this is too difficult you can sit on a chair. You can close your eyes, or keep them open if you prefer.

2. Begin to breathe deeply, and start to notice your breath. Is it deep and slow? Or quick and shallow? Just notice – don't try to change it.

3. Then, as you breathe in, let your hands float upwards, palms up, for the length of the breath.

4. As you breathe out, turn the palms down, and let your hands float back down to your lap.

5. Continue doing this gentle movement with the breath. If your mind wanders, and you start thinking about other things, come back to the breath, and the movement of your hands.

You can do this with music too, but only if it doesn't distract you. And once you can stay with the breath, you can have some fun. Liz likes to bring in her own arm and hand movements that she thinks still create balance but that also encourage a zest for life.

● ● ● ● ● ● ● ● ● ● ● ● ● ● ● ● ● ● ●

FLAMENCO GESTURE

When your hands are up, as you breathe out, let the tip of your thumb and third finger touch, rotate your wrist and flick out the fingers like the Spanish Flamenco dancers.

● ● ● ● ● ● ● ● ● ● ● ● ● ● ● ● ● ● ●

MIST RISING, SNOW FALLING

The first breath here is as above, so that when you breathe out, your palms sweep down like a paintbrush. Then, on the second breath in, open your fingers like the petals of a flower. As you breathe out, bring them together like a closed cluster flower-bud. Repeat this sequence with the paintbrush palms, followed by the opening and closing flower hands.

Whatever your choice, we offer thanks and inspiration to the carers who give so much to the children and young people who need it most. And we end by reminding you how important it is to be kind to yourself, with Liz's Loving Kindness meditation, or *metta*, which you can use at the times you need it most:

> *'May I be well,*
> *May I be happy,*
> *May I be free from suffering.'*

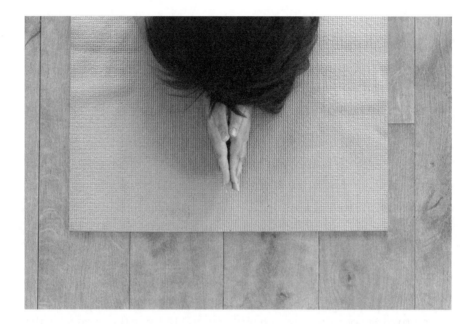

INDEX